Doctors' Secrets

The Road to Longevity

For Kelly,
best wishes,

Canadian Cataloguing in Publication Data

White, Philip A., 1945-
    Doctors' secrets: the road to longevity

Includes bibliographical references and index.
ISBN 0-9689877-0-2

      1. Health. 2. Medicine, preventive. 3. Longevity.
I. McLeod, Donald M., 1953-   II. Heatherington, W.M. III. Title

RA776.75W49 2000   **613**   **C00-901537-X**

Cover photo by Theo Wagner Foto Studio / Invent Ad Communications

Dedication

To our wonderful mothers, Joan McLeod and Evelyn White, whose longevity hormones have allowed them to continue guiding us through life's difficult journey.

CONTENTS

DISCLAIMER

The contents of this book are the opinions of the authors and may not represent the consensus of opinion of the medical profession at this time. The contents of this book are not intended to be used to treat, cure, mitigate or diagnose any medical condition. The readers should consult their doctors before embarking on any changes that could affect their health.

But wherefore do not you a mightier way
Make war upon this bloody tyrant time,
And fortify yourself in your decay
With means more blessed than my barren rhyme?

–William Shakespeare (lived 52 years)

SECTION I

Introduction

A NEW AGE COMING

The event of September 11, 2001, have brought us all closer to our own mortality. For all of those that perished in that terrible tragedy our thoughts are with you and your families. For those that live on, our heightened awareness of how precious life is will always be a memorial to you.

With that in mind, we realise that we are at the threshold of a new era, a new age. By this the authors are not referring to future exploits in space. Nor are we thinking of the coming marvels in computers. Rather, what we see before us is much more astounding than almost anything you can imagine. And more important.

What lies before us is nothing short of a revolution, a revolution that takes place not in society or in world government, but within our own bodies. We are now at the threshold of halting, and even reversing, the aging process. We are at the point where we can now, turn back the clock.

As important as discoveries in space travel or computers may be, there are none that can compare to the revolution taking place in the field of anti-aging. We may, in the future, marvel at rockets going to Mars, or look wide-eyed with wonder at how a computer can operate an entire factory, but if we are bedridden with age, or stuck in a wheelchair with decaying bones, or hobbling painfully on two canes, all of these marvels will lose their luster. For, who amongst us, as we reach our declining years, would not trade any of these marvels for the chance to walk as sprightly at 80 as we did at 40? To maintain a lean and muscled body into what was formerly thought of as "old age"?

Of course, to 20 year olds of today, this prospect is not such a big deal. They, like ourselves at 20, feel they will live forever. But at 40 or 50, this outlook will change. Once the middle age decline sets in, they will then come to value most highly this revolution in anti-aging therapies. And revolutionary these new therapies are.

Turning Back the Clock

In the past we have all been subject to the inevitable creep of aging: the wrinkles, the aches and pains, the battle of the bulge, the loss of vigor, and so on. Now, for the first time, we possess the means of halting these scourges, of halting the aging process itself, and of greatly extending the human life span.

In the past there have been various anti-aging therapies - vitamins, ginseng, ginkgo biloba, etc.. And although many of these therapies may be efficacious in girding our defenses against aging, it is only recently that treatments have been discovered that can help to stop aging in its tracks.

The most recent and most amazing of these involve Human Growth Hormone replacement therapy. Just some of the benefits shown to be conferred by this therapy are:

- gains in muscle mass
- losses of fatty tissue
- restoration of potent sexual function
- restoration of youthful energy

So effective has Human Growth Hormone replacement therapy shown itself to be, that once it becomes widely available we may well consider that we have embarked on a new era, a new age. Controversy at the Australian 2000 Olympics demonstrated that Human Growth Hormone (HGH) is a powerful fitness enhancer, and with the use of HGH, we are now able to start the process of turning back the clock. For many of us, HGH therapy will likely turn back the clock a decade or two. Add one or two other minor measures and we can probably make that a gain of two or three decades. Which will then take us to future discoveries that will extend our lives still further. And on and on.

So we invite you to join us in the pages ahead, as we embark upon a new path, a new road - the road to longevity.

Remember, that the views that we express are those shared by *"Anti-aging"* Doctors.

"Antiaging and Somapause treatments" are not covered by regular medical plans, as aging is not accepted by private or publicly funded systems as a medical problem or a disease process.

AN OVERVIEW

The Aging Process

From earliest times human beings have looked with dismay at the aging process. We have seen crows feet claw their way around the eyes of our grandparents, and then our parents. We have seen the wrinkles invade, first as faint lines, then as fissures in cheek and forehead, and finally as ugly furrows cutting down into lips that had once been smooth and beautiful.

We have seen bodies which had once been hard and sculpted turn to flab, then sag and fold, eventually becoming hunched and bowed in their ultimate obeisance to gravity.

And we have seen, in the latter stages of aging, bodies withered, skin hanging over bone; faces lined like road maps; eyes of dull staring where a bright twinkle had once been, sunk deep and dark in their sockets.

And the earth beckoned.

And now we, the baby boomers who came of age in the sixties and seventies, are finally hitting our 40's and 50's. We, who thought 30 was old and who reveled in Bob Dylan's tune "Forever Young", are now finding we are no longer young. And now we, after the passage of these 20 or 30 years, are beginning to see those signs of aging in ourselves.

We see a plumper face staring back in the mirror these days, with some puffiness under the eyes, a few faint lines here and there. And sometimes when we bend over to pick something up there is a barely perceptible grunt that escapes the throat as we stand up again. And when we get out of the car after riding around for an hour or two we feel a stiffness in the joints that's never been there before. And at the beach or poolside we spend more time lolling in the sun, less time frolicking in the water.

So now, after decades of supposed indestructibility, we are finally coming to the realization that, as it was for our parents and grandparents before us, so it is for us now: it is our turn - our turn for the aging process. And worst of all, we can do nothing about it, nothing to stave it off. Or can we?

The Impossible Dream

From time immemorial we have dreamt of becoming immortal. That was, of course, impossible, but the dream was always there.

In the dark ages alchemists sought to transmute base metals into gold, wizards sought to find the elixir of life, a potion that would allow us to live forever. But for centuries the dream eluded the dreamer.

Finally, around the middle of the last century, nuclear physicists did manage to transmute some elements into others. Most notable amongst these was the transmutation of hydrogen into helium - and the hydrogen bomb. But the means of staving off aging still eluded us.

Now, at the beginning of the 21st Century, all this is about to change. Recent discoveries into the aging process are about to usher us through a new portal, a portal which may well take us through the aging process without the usual burden of decrepitude and decay: the portal that ushers us onto the road to longevity.

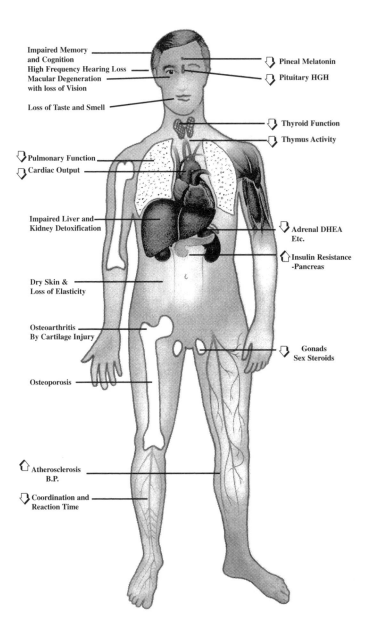

Impaired Memory and Cognition
High Frequency Hearing Loss
Macular Degeneration with loss of Vision

Loss of Taste and Smell

Pineal Melatonin
Pituitary HGH

Thyroid Function
Thymus Activity

Pulmonary Function
Cardiac Output

Impaired Liver and Kidney Detoxification

Adrenal DHEA Etc.
Insulin Resistance -Pancreas

Dry Skin & Loss of Elasticity

Osteoarthritis By Cartilage Injury

Gonads Sex Steroids

Osteoporosis

Atherosclerosis B.P.

Coordination and Reaction Time

Biological Aging

Life Span

Since the days of the cave man our human life span has grown steadily longer. Agriculture, once invented, provided a more dependable food supply. And a steadier, less nomadic existence. All of which, no doubt, conferred a greater chance of living longer. In addition, it set the stage for still further development - new tools and new ways of doing things over the centuries that would make life easier.

Some inventions come immediately to mind: the steam engine, for example. It allowed us to haul loads that previously were unthinkable. Other inventions are not as obvious. Central heating, for instance, which took a lot of the dampness and chill out of everyday living. Or the flush toilet, which conferred new levels of sanitation. All of these inventions, and countless others over the centuries, undoubtedly added years to the average person's life.

But it is in the last two hundred years that the average life span has made its greatest gains. Around the early 1700's the average life expectancy in America was about 25 years of age. By the year 1900, however, the average life span had increased to around 48 years. Now, in the year 2000, the average American can expect to reach almost to the age of 80. And although women still outlive men in most societies, we, at last, have some answers to this puzzle as well.

It is in the realm of science and medicine, especially during the past century, where the greatest gains in longevity were made: insulin; penicillin and the antibiotics which followed; advances in surgical techniques. All have added years and decades to lives that would otherwise have been cut short. Very few questioned the benefits of these life extending discoveries.

What all of this means, however, is that most of us today can expect to live on into ripe old age - with the attendant aches and pains, as well as the increasing decrepitude and decay.

At least that was the case until recent years.

Strengthening Life, Lengthening Life

Although most discoveries in medicine have helped increase the human life span, few have diminished the ravages of aging. Until the last decade or so.

During this period medicine has discovered a number of new treatments that promise to not only extend the human life span, but also to maintain that extension at a youthful, vigorous level. It is now possible to strengthen life and lengthen life.

Some of these new therapies involve the use of nutritional supplements that assist the body in countering particular physiological aspects of aging. Certain vitamins, for example, act as anti-oxidants in the body, thereby combating the oxidizing free radicals that harm body tissue.

More remarkable are the recently employed hormone replacement therapies. These involve restoring to youthful levels hormones such as estrogen, testosterone, progesterone, DHEA, and melatonin, all of which have produced excellent results in countering some aspects of the aging process.

But pre-eminent amongst the new therapies is that which was emphasized in the introduction: Human Growth Hormone replacement therapy. Although the existence of Human Growth Hormone, or HGH, has been known for some time, its full potential - particularly its potential in countering the aging process - has only been looked into and confirmed in the last decade.

The results of HGH replacement therapy are nothing short of astounding. Not only do HGH treatments counter the effects of aging, they are also capable of reversing many of them. Experiments have consistently borne out the favorable results mentioned in the introduction: wrinkles gone or much diminished; fat tissue diminished; muscle mass increased; performance and libido increased in men; libido increased in women. And these are just a few of the positive benefits of this therapy.

In future chapters we will explore in detail all the benefits of HGH, and other therapies as well. We will also look at avenues of current research, and the discoveries that they will likely bring in the near future. And we will explore where these discoveries will probably take us over the next decade, and what they will mean to us by way of extending the human life span still further. We will even consider what the future holds by way of attaining that impossible dream: the dream of living forever!

For now it is enough to say that the most recently discovered therapies, particularly HGH replacement, have the capacity to thwart and retard - The aging process. And to reverse much of it as well.

SECTION II

Aging

Growing Old

What is it to grow old?
Is it to lose the glory of the form,
The luster of the eye?
Is it for beauty to forego her wreath?
—Yes, but not this alone.

Is it to feel our strength—
Not our bloom only but our strength—decay?
Is it to feel each limb
Grow stiffer, every function less exact,
Each nerve more loosely strung?

Yes, this, and more; but not
Ah, 'tis not what in youth we dreamed 'twould be!
'Tis not to have our life
Mellowed and softened as with sunset glow,
A golden day's decline...

It is—last stage of all—
When we are frozen up within, and quite
The phantom of ourselves,
To hear the world applaud the hollow ghost
Which blamed the living man.
    – Matthew Arnold (lived 66 years)

"Age only matters when one is aging."
    – Pablo Picasso (lived 92 years)

"I feel age like an icicle down my back."
    – Dyson Carter

"Old age is an island surrounded by death."
    – Juan Montalvo

Aging

GROWING OLD

"All would live long, but none would be old." So wrote Benjamin Franklin over 200 years ago. It was he, also, who wrote "In this world nothing is certain but death and taxes."

Now, we all know why there are taxes. Sort of. As for death, and its precursor, aging, we - as a species - have never really looked into it. For thousands of years human beings have accepted as inevitable the decline of our latter years, and our ultimate demise. It's the way things were. Our fate.

And still, the question is there: Why do we age? It is a question fundamental to our existence, and yet it is only recently that we have come to ask it at all. The question is fundamental because aging brings us all to a painful and unwelcome decay. And then our extinction - the end of our earthly existence. And yet for centuries we gave the process of aging little thought at all. To be sure, religions through the ages have considered aging and death. But in general, these considerations were from a metaphysical rather than a physical point of view.

Concerning the physical point of view, aging was regarded as inevitable, as inexorable as death itself. It was the natural culmination of life and we could do nothing to stop it.

With the burgeoning of the biological sciences, particularly in the last forty or fifty years, the process of aging has finally come under close scrutiny. With this scrutiny have come numerous theories of aging, some broad in scope, some less so; some relevant to current research, some less so. Let us look at a few of them.

Theories on Aging

Biogrind

Life is a grind: bone on cartilage; bone on bursa; bone on bone. The biogrind.

We begin life with fluid motion, supple joints. Near the end, all too often, the cartilage becomes worn, the bursa become compressed, and it virtually is bone on bone.

This way of looking at aging is encompassed by the Wear and Tear Theory of aging put forth by Dr. August Weismann in 1982. The theory not only applies to bones and joints, but to the entire body. According to this theory, daily use, and most particularly, abuse and overuse, wears the body out.

We add to the wear and tear each time we jump, bend, reach, move; each time we breathe a molecule of pollution into the lungs; each time we ingest a helping of carcinogens as part of the processed foods we eat. These, and all other bodily processes, take their toll. In essence, as postulated by the Wear and Tear Theory, life is grinding us down. The biogrind.

In general this wear and tear - the biogrind - can be countered to some extent with common sense principles of good health: wholesome food, sufficient sleep, proper (not extreme) exercise. In addition, nutritional supplements can also be effective in staving off the wear and tear conferred on us by the years, and the biogrind.

Biosludge

The Waste Accumulation Theory posits that as we age our cells accumulate more waste products like lipofuscins and spherons than they can ultimately dispose of.

In our younger years our physiology is such that anabolism (constructive metabolism) outstrips catabolism (destructive metabolism). Thus, at the height of our youth we have bone, muscle and other tissue being built up more quickly than it is being broken down. Waste products that result from these processes are easily disposed of by our vigorous, youthful cells and detoxification systems. Later in life, the situation is reversed. The result - there is an eventual accumulation of cellular waste products: biosludge.

There is evidence to support this theory. For example, the cells of the body contain a waste product called lipofuscin, or age pigment. This age pigment occurs in cells as small granules, but the granules grow larger as a person ages. In the skin it is this substance that gives rise to the age spots that start to appear around age 40, and thereafter accompany our advancing years. More damning, lipofuscin is found most commonly in the cells of nerves and in heart muscle, such that brain and heart function deteriorate with time.

Biorust: the Free Radical Theory

The Free Radical Theory of aging was first put forth by Dr. Denham Harman in 1954. Dr. Harman's thesis: "Aging is caused by free radical reactions, which may be caused by the environment, from disease, and intrinsic reactions within the aging process."

The idea that dangerous free radicals were produced by normal human biology was considered unlikely until 1969. It was eventually recognised that superoxide and hydroxyl free radicals were causative factors in many degenerative diseases and also in aging. Consequently, aging is not simply the wearing out of body parts, but results from the accumulated damage done to individual cells by free radicals, resulting in decreased function throughout the body.

The Free Radical Theory of aging involves a bit of chemistry. If we hark back to our high school lessons we will recall how atoms, or ions, carry an electrical charge. Each of these ions seeks to neutralize the charge, and may do so by combining with an atom or ion with an opposite charge. In the case of the positively charged sodium ion and the negatively charged chlorine ion, each is able to neutralize the other's opposite charge by combining to form sodium chloride, common table salt. Until they come together and neutralize one another each is very active, looking for something to react with.

Free radicals are atoms, or groups of atoms, that have an imbalance of electrons. This means that the free radicals need another atom or group of atoms to bond with to become neutralized, and stabilized. This makes a free radical extremely active. As free radicals move through the body, they try to achieve chemical and electrical stability by combining with atoms of various body tissues.

The effect of these free radicals on body tissue might be likened to rust on metal or the browning of a freshly cut apple - a sort of biorust.

In the case of iron rust, oxygen atoms eat away at the metal. In the case of "biorust" free radicals eat away at human tissues, at human cells. Not infrequently, free radicals do contain oxygen, a particular form of oxygen that is in a very active state. They attack tissues and cells by forming bonds with atoms that are part of the cell, tearing them away from their cellular structures, and sometimes setting other charged atoms adrift as well - in essence creating more free radicals. In that case the damage is twofold.

Free radicals may attack various body tissues, including collagen and elastin, which are integral components of the skin. These components keep the skin moist and elastic. It is the action of free radicals within the cell that generates some of the aforementioned lipofuscins, ultimately producing age spots. With the passage of time, as the damage (biorust) from the free radicals becomes pronounced, normal skin comes to take on the feel and appearance of scraped parchment.

Besides attacking the tissues and cells of the skin, free radicals can attack other parts of the body, such as heart and kidney tissue. Further, their activity can interfere with the inner chemistry of the cell, disrupting the DNA and RNA, as well as the synthesis of proteins.

Because the action of these free radicals is chemically that of an oxidant, those substances that have shown themselves to be effective in combating them are referred to as anti-oxidants.

Calorie Restriction Theory

The Calorie Restriction Theory postulates that a diet providing optimal nutrition with a minimum of calories will confer the maximum life span to an individual.

This theory, put forward by Dr. Roy Walford, gerontologist at UCLA Medical School, was confirmed by years of scientific experiments with animals.

In a less scientific way we see this same result corroborated in people all around us. Those who overeat and who are considerably overweight appear to have more difficulties with their health. Statistically this is borne out as well: heavy, overweight individuals are more prone to illness and disease, especially cardiovascular problems, and face a lower life expectancy than someone who is fit. Severe calorie restriction is difficult to follow. An average North American eats 2100 - 2600 cal / day and would have to cut down to 1500 cal / day to achieve optimum caloric intake. To date, results have not shown age reversal to be substantial in humans when calories are restricted.

Order to Disorder Theory

The development of the body from infancy is somewhat akin to the construction of a building. It proceeds in an orderly way as appropriate building materials are moved about and fixed in place. But from maturation onward the similarity ceases, and the body begins to produce more faulty materials - such as free radicals - than it can readily take out of the production line. This would be akin to bricklayers having to use inappropriate sized bricks halfway through the construction of a building. The building would be weakened and its longevity would be compromised.

The faulty materials the body must use after maturation, materials that it must incorporate into itself, cause faults with structures and functions in all tissues and organs. Now, instead of the orderly development that had proceeded from infancy, we have a disorderly development proceeding, and it is this disorderliness at the molecular level that takes us into aging.

Thymic Stimulating Theory

The thymus gland has sometimes been called the gland of youth. That is because it is at its greatest size when we are young. At birth it weighs in at 200-250 grams, and shrinks thereafter until, at around age 60, it weighs a mere three grams.

In the past, the role of the thymus gland was a mystery, a largely unexplored mystery, such that nasty and inexplicable illnesses that even caused death were given the name by physicians of "Status Thymus Lymphaticus." This as little as 45 years ago. However, as interest in aging grew, interest in the thymus gland grew as well.

Research so far suggests that the thymus has a positive effect on the immune system. The immunity from T-lymphocytes, programmed in the thymus, is of primary importance in the fight against viruses and cancer. Also, thymic hormones may affect stimulation and production of neurotransmitters, and as well, other hormones produced by both the brain and the endocrine system. All of which suggests that the thymus very likely plays a significant role in the process of aging.

Cross Linkage Theory

In 1942 Johan Bjorksten hypothesized that cross-linking played an important part in the aging process. This cross-linking took place in proteins such as the collagen protein, which is found in skin, tendons, and ligaments.

The collagen protein resembles the legs of a ladder that has very few rungs between them. In addition, each ladder is bound to those beside it by other rungs - the cross-links. As we age, the immune system is less able to clean the blood of impurities, including excess amounts of glucose molecules. These glucose molecules combine with protein to form advanced glycation end products (AGE's), causing yellowing of the teeth for example, and are able to form further cross-links between the ladders of the collagen proteins. In addition, this process gives rise to free radicals as well.

As the cross-links in collagen proteins become more numerous, they hold adjoining ladder rungs more tightly. This causes the collagenous tissue to shrink, which in turn causes skin to shrink, and become less pliable. Further, these cross-links may impede the movement of nutrient and waste between cells.

Mitochondrial Theory

Mitochondria are minute organelles found within the cells of our bodies inherited from our mothers. They are the power plants of the cell, and as such, produce the energy from ATP needed by the body for its many daily tasks. ATP (Adenosine Triphosphate) is an energy providing molecule derived from ADP (Adenosine Diphosphate) in a process called oxidative phosphorylation, a process whereby ADP picks up an extra phosphate. 100 % of the ATP derived from free fatty acid breakdown, and 95 % of the ATP derived from the metabolism of glucose sugar, takes place in the mitochondria. The chemical cycles the mitochondria employ, besides producing energy, also produce free radicals. Unfortunately, the mitochondria, themselves, are quite vulnerable to damage from free radicals. As the damage to the mitochondria accumulates, the DNA can also become damaged, and the DNA of mitochondria cannot be repaired. Further, evidence to date indicates that accumulated mitochondrial damage can render an individual more susceptible to disease. There are nearly 1000 mitochondria in each liver cell but only 20 mitochondria in each sperm cell. Once the mitochondria are lost in the cell they cannot be replaced hence the increasing fatigue, loss of energy and loss of function of the cells as we lose our mitochondria with age.

Errors And Repairs Theory

According to this theory, the aging process is, at least in part, caused by damage to nuclear DNA, and to the related protein production mechanisms in cells. In actuality, cells do have the capability of repairing nuclear DNA damage of this kind. However, the Errors and Repairs Theory postulates further that repairs are never quite 100 percent.

You might compare these kinds of cellular repairs to repairs done on a car that has been in an accident. Often the superficial damage done to the car is no longer detectable after the repair work is done, but stress tests might very well reveal hidden, unrepaired weaknesses within. And sometimes the signs of the inadequate repair work are only too detectable, with doors or fenders improperly aligned, etc.

Example of DNA damage by losing a purine by hydrolysis reaction.

Just as imperfect repair work done on a car will almost certainly hasten its aging and curtail its life expectancy, so too, current thought holds, imperfect repair work done on damaged DNA will similarly take its toll.

Limited Number of Cell Divisions Theory

If we were to find ourselves in a sealed chamber with all we needed to eat, drink, and breathe, we would still soon expire. Our own waste products - especially the carbon dioxide we exhale - would do us in.

For the cells of the body, a similar situation obtains. They need to have their cellular wastes removed or they too will die. Of course, cells will die in any case, but under good conditions they will (except for brain cells) be constantly replacing themselves through ongoing cell division, albeit at a different rate in different structures.

Obviously, then, if the cells of the body could undergo cell division indefinitely, we might contemplate a much expanded life span, with fewer age-related problems.

As an experiment, a French surgeon, Dr. Alexis Carrel, immersed pieces of a chicken heart in a saline solution, a solution that contained various minerals in the same concentration as found in chicken blood. He disposed of the waste products daily, and was able to keep the cells of the chicken heart alive for 28 years. Needless to say, that was well beyond the life span of any ordinary chicken.

Now, it is obvious that, while most of us would love to have our bodies live on well past the normal life span, we would not wish to achieve this objective at the expense of living in a saline solution, in a giant petri dish, in pieces.

Not to worry, that will not be recommended. As it turns out, the success of Dr. Carrel's experiment lay partly in the fact that fresh cells had been inadvertently added to the culture that was keeping the heart cells alive.

However, the experiment does explain why the cells of an older person, which contain more waste products, divide more slowly and fewer times than do cells from an embryo that are less burdened with waste.

The Hayflick Limit Theory

One of the most important discoveries in cellular biology, a discovery equally important in our under-standing of the aging process, was made in 1961. The discovery was made by two cell biologists, Dr. Hayflick and Dr. Moorehead, and it involved an experiment that demonstrated the senescence, or aging, of cells.

Dr. Hayflick had postulated that the aging process was determined by a biological clock that existed in every living cell.

The two scientists, carried out experiments somewhat along the lines of Dr. Carrel's experiment, using fibroblast cells (found in lung, skin, muscle, and heart tissue). These experiments demonstrated conclusively that the life span of a cell is limited. It could divide approximately 50 times over a period of years, at which point it ceased dividing.

The rate at which these cell divisions took place appeared to be governed by the amount of nutrient available. Cells that had an oversupply of nutrient completed the 50 cell divisions in about a year. Cells that had an under supply of nutrient took three times longer than did normal cells to complete their 50 divisions. While going through this division process, some cells went through changes and degenerated prior to reaching the 50 cell division limit. The parts of the cell most affected by the degenerative process were the cell organelles (like mitochondria), membranes, and genetic material (like DNA).

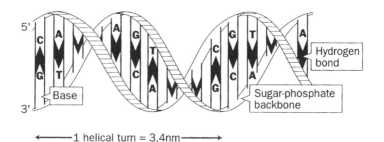

←————1 helical turn = 3.4nm————→

Part of DNA strand showing bonds and Double Helix with bases A,T,C,G. (Adenine, Thymine, Cytosine, Guanine)

Given the degeneration that befalls some cells, and their eventual loss in organs and tissues, it is a very reasonable conclusion that this loss plays a large part in the aging process.

The Telomerase Theory of Aging

The field of research dealing with telomeres and telomerase is one of the most exciting fields in the quest to defeat the aging process.

Telomeres are lengths of nucleic acids (DNA) that extend from the tip of our 46 chromosomes. They have been described as resembling the plastic tips on the ends of shoelaces.

As the cells in our bodies divide, the chromosomes inside the nucleus divide as well. With each division the telomeres on the ends of each chromosome become shortened. After a certain number of cell divisions these telomeres have been reduced to but a fraction of their original length. At this point the cell ceases to divide further. It becomes senescent and eventually dies. This suggests most strongly that the telomere is the biological clock that governs a cell's ability to divide, the regulator or counter that is responsible for finally halting cell division: the previously invisible hand behind the Hayflick Limit.

The telomeres, in turn, have their length determined by an enzyme called telomerase. And the production of telomerase, finally, is regulated by the telomerase gene and Human Growth Hormone may activate this gene to prevent telomere shortening.

In youthful cells there is more telomerase present,

actively preserving the length of the telomeres as these cells divide. In older cells, the levels of telomerase is lower, and at this stage more of the telomere is lost with each division.

The latest research to date shows that by maintaining high, youthful levels of telomerase in a cell we confer upon the cell the capacity to go on dividing indefinitely.

Conversely, where the telomeres have become shortened, the diminished capacity of a cell to divide shows up in the form of wrinkled skin, or hair loss. Scientists at Geron Corporation in San Francisco have been doing research with telomerase for many years. In mice, genetically engineered to have short telomeres, some accompanying aspects of aging are also present. In a disease called Dyskeratosis Congenita, where shortened telomeres occur as well, there are also conditions present that often accompany aging: anemia, poor skin and nails, and proneness to infection. All of this suggests that a shortening of the telomeres has a direct connection with aging.

And this is where the excitement in present day research lies: find a way to keep the levels of telomerase in our cells elevated, and the cells should continue to divide in their original, youthful manner, avoiding senescence; keep the cells youthful in the various organs and tissues, and the organs and tissues remain youthful and healthy; keep the organs and tissues youthful and healthy and we remain youthful and healthy.

So the research race is on. But the road to success is not without its pitfalls. For one, telomerase, while found at high levels in youthful cells, is also found - as one might expect - at high levels in cancer cells: no doubt the reason cancer cells are able to continue their cell divisions in a rampant manner, although this is more likely an effect rather than a cause phenomenon. On the other hand, this fact may eventually lead cancer research to a new and formidable weapon in the war against that deadly disease.

In the war on aging, research on telomerase is proceeding apace, particularly in the field of genetics. As for affecting telomerase levels by means of hormonal therapies, researchers have already arrived at programs that are bearing fruit. More on these hopeful topics in future chapters.

Good News Coming

We have examined but a handful of the theories of aging that have been put forth over the years. Until recently, no single theory has held sway throughout.

CIRCLE OF AGING

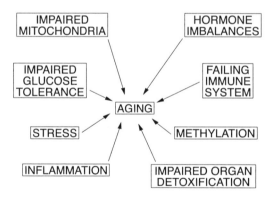

Some have described the effects of aging, or have set forth intermediate causes or partial causes, rather than a major, elementary cause. Some may have spoken accurately to parts of the puzzle, but not all of it. Some, like the Wear and Tear theory, are very broad in their hypotheses. and consequently, suggest little by way of future therapy, or research direction. The telomerase theory may be changing that, for it is very specific and offers a very pointed direction as to future therapy and future research.

We have seen many important discoveries made in the past two decades, but many still lie ahead. It belongs to the future to sort it all out. For the present, we - the baby boomers - have anti-aging therapies available to us many of which were completely unknown ten or fifteen years ago. For the first time ever we have the means at hand to virtually halt some aspects of aging in its tracks. For the first time ever scientists - not charlatans or wool gatherers but realistic scientists- are talking about defeating the aging process totally, are talking about human beings living forever, are talking about - immortality!

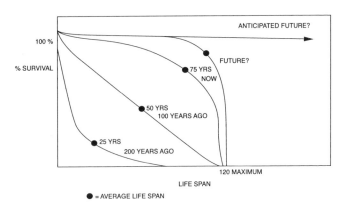

New Treatments for longevity, like Telomerase Therapy, may make immortality possible.

If much in the foregoing pages has been somber and gloomy - aging and death are rarely light topics - almost all that is before us in the coming pages is about good news. Much of this good news involves the hormone replacement therapies, and the most striking and exciting of these right now, involves Human Growth Hormone.

"His days shall be 120 years." The Holy Bible, Genesis VI, vs 3.

Notes

<u>SECTION III</u>

HGH: Human Growth Hormone

"The fountain of youth lies within the cells of each of us. All you need to do is release it."

– Dr. Ronald Klatz

"Envision HGH as a master key to a building. The master key not only unlocks the main door, but it can unlock every other door in the building... By opening all doors, HGH allows in refreshing, invigorating and rejuvenating influences that revive each organ in the body."

– Dr. Edmund Chein

"The overall deterioration that comes with growing old is not inevitable. We now realize that some aspects of it can be prevented or reversed."

– Dr. Daniel Rudman

"GH is essential for normal adult life and without it, life expectancy is shortened, energy and vitality reduced and the quality of life is impaired. The medical case for GH replacement is now proven beyond any reasonable medical and scientific doubt."

– Peter Sonksen,
GH and IGF Research Journal '98

Doctors' Secrets

HGH: The Master Hormone

THE TIME MACHINE

You feel yourself waking slowly. Eyes half open, you stretch your arms, your legs. It feels good. Something so simple as stretching and it feels so good. You open your eyes all the way and see the light streaming through the window. The morning is calling you. You slip your feet over the side of the bed, stretch your arms once more for that good feeling, and then spring to your feet. So many things before you: perhaps a jog through the park; a long walk down by the river; or maybe down to the courts for some tennis, and then a good swim afterwards. Perhaps all of it. For the day is yours to move through....

Can you remember mornings like that? The eagerness, the anticipation? The body moving fluidly, effortlessly, painlessly? When you could take on a day that had no limits? Or at least it felt that way?

For most of us in our forties and fifties, that kind of easy-moving body is no longer with us. And some of that lively, eager attitude has probably faded a bit as well.

And yet...how good it would be to have those days back, that vigorous young body back, that alacrity of spirit back. To hop into an H. G. Wells' kind of time machine and get it all back.

Alas, those days are gone, faded into the mists of time, and we will never bring them back. There is no time machine.

Or is there?

In reality, although we have not the means to travel back in time, we **do** have the means of bringing our younger, stronger bodies back, back to us here and now in the present. Back from how they were ten, fifteen, twenty years ago. So we do, in a sense, have a time machine. And that time machine is called somatotropin, or Human Growth Hormone, **HGH**.

The Modern Miracle

Suppose someone were to tell you there was a simple way to:

- Increase muscle mass and lose fat, without dieting or exercising.
- Increase bone mass and reverse the process leading to osteoporosis.
- Increase the thickness and elasticity of the skin, and improve skin tone.
- Improve cardiac function.
- Improve kidney function.
- Strengthen the immune system.
- Recharge sexual desire and performance.
- Speed the healing of wounds.
- Lower blood pressure and cholesterol levels.
- Promote regeneration of aged and weakened organs such as kidneys, liver, heart.
- Diminish or eliminate wrinkles.
- Improve cartilage formation in joints.

- Replenish youthful energy levels, improve aerobic capacity.
- Regain youthful exuberance and improved outlook.
- Achieve better and more restful sleep.
- Diminish or eliminate cellulite.
- Regrow hair (in some cases) or reduce the gray.

You would say this was a miracle. You would say that no single substance could do all that. That it was impossible.

And you'd be wrong!

Human Growth Hormone - HGH - has been shown to do all of that. HGH is the modern miracle. It is here now and it works. The data of the past few decades, particularly the last decade, confirms the amazing, anti-aging effects of HGH. And the data continues to amass, further corroborating the previous studies.

What is HGH?

What is this amazing substance, HGH? As its full name suggests, HGH is a hormone. Ernest Starling coined the term "hormone" in his paper, "On the chemical correlation of the functions of the body" in 1905.

A hormone is a substance made in one part of the body that can affect the activity of cells in another part of the body, sometimes even in a remote part of the body. In a way, hormones are like messengers, carrying a message from a gland, for example, to other cells of the body, instructing them to effect a particular activity. In the case of HGH, as long as the levels are not excessive, the message is all good news.

HGH is produced in the **anterior** pituitary gland, which is located at the base and towards the center of the brain, back in behind the eyes. The pituitary is one of the endocrine glands, which means it secretes its "message" directly into the bloodstream.

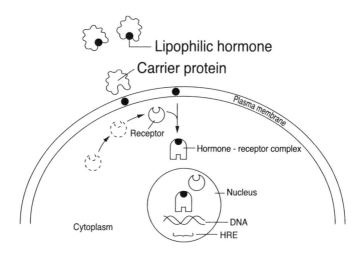

Hormones leave the carrier protein at the cell surface to attach to a receptor that subsequently instructs the DNA to produce protein.

Once HGH is released into the bloodstream, much of it attaches to receptors on the liver and instructs it to produce a protein called Insulin-Like Growth Factor-1 (IGF-1). It is in this form that HGH does much of its work. Both HGH and IGF-1 have receptor activity on our cells. Much of our IGF-1 attaches to binding proteins of which there are several, and each of these combinations have effects on cell function. It is by attaching to the appropriate receptor sites at cells throughout the body that HGH and IGF-1 bring about their anti-aging effects.

The gene for HGH is on the long arm of chromosome 17 in a cluster of five genes, while that for IGF-1 is on the long arm of chromosome 12.

HGH History and Development

HGH was discovered in the 1920's, and was thereafter largely ignored.

In the late 1950's HGH resurfaced. Endocrinologist Maurice Rabin, at the New England Medical Center in Boston, Massachusetts, began treating a growth stunted child with injections of HGH. The child, whose body was not able to produce its own HGH, then resumed growing. This pioneering work of Dr. Rabin's set the stage for HGH. More doctors began employing this therapy to treat children with growth deficiencies, with the same wonderful result. Then came some tragic news.

The HGH used to treat these children had been obtained from Africa, extracted from the brains of cadavers. Unhappily, the process by which the hormone was extracted from the pituitaries in these brains, also extracted an element which had previously infected some of these brains. It was the Prion that caused Creutzfeldt-Jacob disease. And it was this hitch-hiking Prion that led to the tragedy, just as a similar element led to the "mad cow disease" controversy in Europe.

During the 1950's in the U.S. seven children of the 5,000 who had undergone this HGH extraction treatment contracted Creutzfeldt-Jacob disease. The expected incidence would have been from 1: 100,000 to 1: 1,000,000. The treatments were discontinued and the FDA banned the use of this extraction.

It is, however, rarely an ill wind that blows no good at all. With the benefits of HGH already apparent, and with the original source of HGH lost, drug companies were spurred on to find a way of synthesizing HGH in the lab. Given the potential benefits of HGH, with even more being foreshadowed, the U.S. government offered incentives to this end.

Recombinant HGH

Producing HGH in the lab would prove to be a daunting task. Hormones are made up of proteins; proteins, in turn, are made up of amino acids. In the case of HGH, the chain that makes up its protein consists of 191 amino acids strung together. Imagine having to string 191 various kinds of beads together in a row, getting them on the string in a specific order, without making a single mistake. Then try and imagine doing this at the molecular level and you get something of the idea of the difficulties involved.

It was a challenge well suited to a company called Genentech, co-founded by Nobel prize winner, Herbert Boyer, who also played a major role in the development of genetic engineering. The task was assigned to David Goeddel, one of Genentech's leading scientists. Employing the techniques of gene splicing, Goeddel's team was able, after a year of intense work, to clone the HGH molecule - almost. What they ended up with was a molecule that did everything that HGH did, but was short by one amino acid.

During this same period drug manufacturer Eli Lily had been working on the problem of replicating HGH as well. Within a year of Goeddel's success, a team at Eli Lily were able to complete the task down to the final amino acid, producing the entire HGH molecule with all 191 amino acids. Ultimately, both companies were awarded the right to produce and distribute HGH. One company could make HGH with the help of E. Coli bacteria, and the other company could make HGH from mammalian cells with the use of recombinant DNA technology.

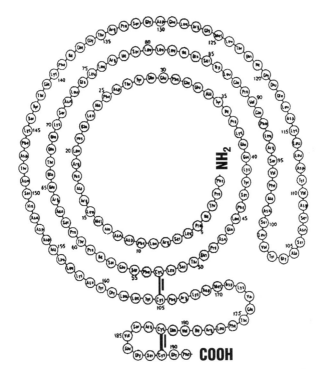

191 Amino Acids of Human Growth Hormone with two Disulfide bridges.

The most important point, however, was that scientists, and the medical community, now had a totally pure source of HGH, a source which provided HGH that was in every way like the HGH produced in the human body - right down to the final atom. Just as a molecule of salt you might make in a high school lab by combining sodium and chlorine would be identical to a molecule of salt produced by the body in perspiration, so too a molecule of HGH that could now be produced in the lab was identical to a molecule of HGH produced by the body. The procedure might be infinitely more complex, but now at least it was possible.

The upshot was that finally a new, safe, supply of HGH would be forthcoming, that treatments for children with growth defects could be resumed. Important as that was, yet a more widespread and far-reaching application for HGH was about to unfold. A second breakthrough, this time in the war on aging, was at hand. This breakthrough would be brought forth by an endocrinologist working in Madison, Wisconsin, Dr. Daniel Rudman.

The Rudman Study

Dr. Rudman had come to the conclusion that since hormonal production and activity decline in the human body as we begin to age, perhaps this decline was involved in the aging process. At the forefront of this hormonal decline, Dr. Rudman concluded, was HGH. The production of HGH in the body begins to drop off sharply around age 25, about the same time that the physical decline begins to set in. In addition, the results of studies in Denmark and Sweden employing genetically engineered HGH that had newly become available, offered indirect support for Dr. Rudman's hypothesis.

In these studies, children and adults with HGH deficiencies due to pituitary malfunction, were given injections of HGH. Thereafter these individuals, in whom some wasting of body tissue had occurred, attained a more normal lean body mass. Now, one of the most obvious signs of aging is the decline of lean body tissue - our muscles become less pronounced, our bones less dense; also, we tend to pack on more fat. Dr. Rudman's intriguing idea was this: What would happen if HGH were to be given to individuals who were aging but were otherwise normal and healthy?

To answer this question, Dr. Rudman recruited 26 men ranging in age from 61 to 80. All exhibited the characteristic bodies of those in their advancing years: the loss of firm, well defined muscles, and that extra cushion of fat around the middle: the amorphous rotundity of age.

A few men dropped out of the study, but of the 21 men who completed it, 12 were given HGH injection throughout while 9 in the control group received no treatment.

All had been directed to continue on through the study with their lifestyles unchanged, to do nothing different or out of the ordinary - smoke if they smoked previously, drink if they drank previously, and take exercise only to the extent they had taken exercise previously. Alter nothing in their normal patterns of behavior.

The results of this study were unmistakable. Those who had been administered HGH over the six month period had an average 8.8% gain in muscle mass, a 14% decrease in fat. Their skin had grown thicker and the vertebrae of the lower spine had increased in bone mass. By Dr. Rudman's evaluation they had dropped 10 to 20 years of aging from their physical makeup. In essence, they had turned back the clock, their bodies appeared to be 10 or 20 years younger.

This remarkable result was immediately recognized as a stunning breakthrough in the war on aging. Dr. Rudman was excited about the results and was eager to run future tests and experiments. Unhappily, he never got the chance. He died from a pulmonary embolism in 1994. But he had shown the way. And now, at the beginning of the new millennium, the field of anti-aging is burgeoning. New, positive data keeps flowing in.

HGH Side Effects

It may be that one day a super potion or a super drug will be discovered that has no side effects whatsoever. But that day is not yet and not now. However, HGH does come close when used properly.

For all the benefits HGH conferred on individuals in the Rudman experiment, it did also manifest a tendency to bring on some unwanted side effects, the main two being carpal tunnel syndrome (a painful condition of the wrist) and gynecomastia (enlarged breasts). Later studies have shown that these side effects can be virtually eliminated - while at the same time retaining the benefits - by giving smaller amounts more frequently, than had been administered by Dr. Rudman.

A very different application of HGH, treatments administered by Dr. Robert Kerr in San Gabriel, California, also produced a host of positive results. In this case, Dr. Kerr had prescribed HGH to numerous patients in his family practice, many of whom were youthful athletes and bodybuilders, and all of whom were already in good physical condition. Yet even here, where there was much less room for improvement, excellent results were achieved, particularly with strong gains in muscle mass, and significant losses of fat.

But there was a down side and some of these patients reported some side effects. Again, at this point in HGH research, little was known concerning dosages, or appropriate circumstances in which HGH should be prescribed. Many of the patients in this case were young and healthy to begin with, having youthful high levels of HGH as part of their normal physiology. To receive further high doses on top of that was almost certainly the reason those side effects manifested themselves. Again, to emphasize the point, these dosages were administered when data on HGH was being worked out largely by trial and error. Since then, much data in this area has been amassed, and study after study since have turned up results indicating that with proper dosages and schedules, administered to the appropriate individuals, side effects have been virtually reduced to zero.

One study in particular that underscored this point was a study conducted by Maxine Papadakis and colleagues at the University of California in San Francisco. In that study, the same doses of HGH used by Dr. Rudman in his initial study were administered. Similar side effects ensued, including joint pain and swelling. When the dose was reduced by approximately 50%, the side effects abated sharply or ceased altogether within two weeks of the dose being reduced - but the benefits were maintained.

It would not be an understatement to say that with current knowledge concerning HGH and dosage, side effects should now - except for rare instances - be a thing of the past.

Other Studies And Experiments

Although Dr. Rudman's study was pivotal in demonstrating the formidable power of HGH in combating the aging process, there have been other studies as well. Some have focused on one area, some on another.

In Europe, there have been studies by Professor Peter Sonksen at St. Thomas' Hospital Medical School in London, Dr. Jens Sandahl Christiansen at the University of Aarhus in Denmark, and Dr. Bengt-Ake Bengtssön at the University of Göteborg in Sweden. These studies have largely been concerned with HGH deficiencies in adults caused by pituitary disease.

Many of these patients exhibited symptoms not that dissimilar from the characteristic conditions associated with aging, the most obvious being the wasting away of muscle tissue and the bulbous, ill-defined body shape. The consequences of employing HGH replacement therapy in these studies have been very favorable. In the words of Dr. Sonksen, they have given "...remarkably consistent results."

Thomas Falkheden, a Swedish scientist describing the condition of patients who had undergone the removal of the pituitary gland, included symptoms such as a lower basal metabolism, impaired heart and kidney function, reduced blood volume - all conditions which make a regular appearance in the aged. Further, these conditions were present in those patients despite the fact that most of them were undergoing appropriate hormone replacement therapy, with one glaring exception - they were not receiving HGH. When HGH was included in the replacement therapy, for a great many of these patients, their condition was seen to improve.

Given that HGH replacement therapy has demonstrated a significant effectiveness in ameliorating many of the aging-like effects induced by pituitary removal, it is not surprising that experimenters like Dr. Rudman should find it effective as an anti-aging agent.

One thing we should bear in mind about the studies on both pituitary removal and aging, is that these are real, live, flesh-and-blood people behind all the graphs and statistics. And with all the positive results accruing to the HGH studies now ongoing, that it is real, live people - not lifeless numbers and statistics - who are being helped.

By way of illustration: One such person in Dr. Bengtsson's care, a young man around the age of twenty, first came to the hospital in a very lethargic state. He had, for most of his life, been a loner, overweight and miserable, and had previously spent his days in idle depression. He came to the hospital with the specific intention of being certified for a disability pension. It was determined that HGH therapy might improve his condition and he agreed to undergo treatment.

The transformation that resulted was striking. The young man lost flab and trimmed down, acquired a newfound energy and enthusiasm for life - and a girlfriend as well. The change was so complete that when he offered his photo ID to a sales clerk at a liquor store, bearing a picture of his former self, the clerk refused to accept it. She could not believe that it was a photo of the same man standing before her.

Such is the case for all the numbers and statistics presented here in this book. Although the use of numbers, graphs, and statistics allows a greater scientific perception of what is happening in certain situations, establishing causal relationships and the like, we must never forget that these numbers represent real people. And as is becoming more and more apparent in the case of HGH replacement therapy, it is real people whose lives are being revitalized and transformed in a way previously thought impossible.

Two Personal Histories

Undoubtedly, the most extensive study and the most comprehensive data concerning HGH has come about from the efforts of two men, Dr. Edmund Chein, and Dr. Leon Cass Terry, from the Palm Springs Life Extension Institute and the University of Wisconsin, respectively.

Both men came to their involvement with HGH via personal experience.

In the case of Dr. Chein, that personal experience began with chest pains in his out of shape body. He had a pot belly, high levels of cholesterol and triglycerides, and a partially blocked coronary artery. In Dr. Chein's words: "I was aging, I was in pain, and my cardiologist warned me to cut back on work or risk devastating health problems." His cardiologist also suggested he go on medication that would lower his cholesterol.

Dr. Chein, who had been working with patients recovering from injuries that had also damaged various glands, saw first hand the beneficial results of hormone replacement therapy. Patients on hormone replacement quickly regained lost energy, endurance, and muscle strength. And although aware of the efficacy of melatonin and DHEA replacement in slowing the process of aging, nothing had impressed him so much as learning about HGH and Dr. Rudman's study. Only with HGH had there been observed effects such as to suggest that the aging process was not only being retarded, but in some aspects, was actually being reversed.

Taking the biblical injunction (Physician, heal thyself) to heart, Dr. Chein embarked on a program of total hormone replacement. Tests had shown that in many instances his hormone levels were low, some extremely so. Dr. Chein reasoned that if he could bring these hormone levels back to what they had been when he was a 20 year old, then the rest of his physiology should follow suit, and his body should self-correct.

His reasoning proved to be right on target. Within six months the chest pains had abated, his cholesterol and triglyceride levels were now normal, and he was even losing his pot belly. He had become a believer.

So strongly convinced was he that hormone replacement was the best way to combat the aging process - especially in the case of HGH - that in 1994 he opened the Palm Springs Life Extension Institute. As he put it "...hormone replacement therapy is the best option open to us today to prevent the diseases and other side effects of aging."

The second personal history is that of neuroendocrinologist and professor of neurology at the Medical College of Wisconsin in Milwaukee, Dr. Leon Cass Terry. His story bears some resemblance to Dr. Chein's. One difference was that for all of his 55 years of age, Dr. Terry had kept in fairly good condition. But, as he says "...my body fat composition, like a lot of older males, had changed. I had gotten that little belt around the middle."

Dr. Terry had been a friend and colleague of Dr. Rudman and the two had begun a pilot project on IGF-1 and neurological disorders. The project, unhappily, was cut short by Dr. Rudman's untimely death. Dr. Terry was, however, eminently aware of the work taking place to combat aging.

When he heard from a friend, who had been a former world class weightlifter, that he was receiving treatment from Dr. Chein, Dr. Terry embarked on a similar course. In less than two months, under Dr. Chein's care, he was achieving extremely good results with HGH replacement therapy. As he states, with an almost palpable exuberance, "I lost a lot of fat with growth hormone. I don't think my energy level has changed because I've always been high energy. But my libido has changed significantly along with my sexual performance. I don't get nearly as winded or exhausted when I work out now. The dumbbell press on which I used to lift 30 pounds, I'm now up to 50 pounds and I can kill it."

From 1995 through 1996, Dr. Chein and Dr. Terry were in fruitful collaboration. During that time, working with hundreds of patients at the Palm Springs Life Extension Institute, they amassed a mountain of data. All of it good.

Palm Springs Data

Benjamin Disraeli once said, "There are three kinds of lies: lies, damned lies, and statistics." Obviously he liked statistics no more than the average person does today. But where statistics are properly employed they can be extremely truthful and useful. And although statistics may dehumanize information, they do convey large quantities of information in a short space. In the case of the information coming out of the Palm Springs Life Extension Institute, these statistics convey a great deal of great information.

The following statistics were obtained from 202 patients who were treated at the Institute from 1994 to 1996.

Strength, Exercise, and Body Fat Improvement (as % of Test Population)

Muscle Strength	88%
Muscle Size	81%
Body Fat Loss	72%
Exercise Tolerance	81%
Exercise Endurance	83%

Skin & Hair

Skin Texture	71%
Skin Thickness	68%
Skin Elasticity	71%
Wrinkle Disappearance	51%
New Hair Growth	38%

Healing, Flexibility & Resistance

Healing of Old Injuries	55%
Healing of Other Injuries	61%
Healing Capacity	71%
Back Flexibility	53%
Resistance to Common Illness	73%

Sexual Function

Sexual Potency	75%
Frequency, Duration of Erection	62%
Frequency of Night Urination	57%
Hot Flashes	58%
Menstrual Cycle Regulation	38%

Energy, Emotions & Memory

Energy level	84%
Emotional Stability	67%
Attitude Toward Life	78%
Memory	62%

These amazing results were achieved by hormone replacement therapy, chief amongst them being HGH. In most cases, the results were attained in one to three months, and improvement continued over the following six months of treatment.

By testing beforehand, the hormonal levels for each patient were determined and a therapy tailored to the particular needs of that patient. By further testing throughout the course of treatment, the hormones requiring replacement could be monitored and dosages adjusted.

Dr. Chein and Dr. Terry tailored their treatments based on the fact that the peak levels of HGH generally occur in men, one to two hours after we first fall asleep at night. During the day the pattern is less predictable, with smaller bursts - or pulses - of HGH showing up in the bloodstream at various times, but always at levels significantly lower than the major rise during early sleep. Women secrete in smaller bursts throughout the 24 hours.

In the initial days of HGH, when children were first being treated for pituitary deficiencies, they were treated in a hospital setting. They were given large doses of HGH three times a week. This was far from ideal and did not produce ideal results. As Dr. Chein has observed, "We are not equipped for or used to handling large doses of HGH only three times a week." He compares this to compelling people to eat only three huge meals per week, rather than three or four smaller meals each day. Consequently, at Palm Springs, HGH treatments are set at a low dose, high frequency schedule.

By "micro-managing" each patient's treatment in this way, and by administering the doses of HGH to mimic the levels that the body naturally attains, the side effects were reduced to a negligible factor. Dr. Chein and Dr. Terry have made HGH replacement a stunning win-win situation.

HGH Physiology

There is a second way in which we can elevate the levels of HGH in the body besides injections, a more natural way. To understand how it works it will be helpful if we first explore just a little of the physiology of HGH in the body.

As we have seen, HGH is produced in the anterior (front) part of the pituitary gland, which is located near the base of the brain, and then released into the bloodstream. Its production and release are largely governed by a number of feedback systems, the most important part of which involves a part of the brain called the hypothalamus. In a stripped down, over-simplified version of how the pituitary and the hypothalamus affect each other, we might regard the hypothalamus (as part of the more complex feedback loop) as a governor to the pituitary.

When levels of HGH in the blood become altered, this is detected by the hypothalamus, which reacts to the change. For example, if levels of HGH have reached what is regarded as maximal by the hypothalamus, the hypothalamus releases a hormone called somatostatin, which tells the pituitary to cut back on the amount of HGH it is releasing. Somatostatin is also known as Growth Hormone Inhibiting Hormone (GHIH), and it is released from the pancreas, thyroid and gut as well. These somatostatin peptides will also inhibit thyroid and pancreas function. When levels of HGH are low, this too is detected by the hypothalamus, which releases another hormone called Growth Hormone Releasing Hormone (GHRH), which in turn instructs the pituitary to release more HGH. Since GHRH pulses regularly over the 24 hour period it is known that GHIH is the true "gatekeeper" for HGH release. GHIH will occasionally drop to low levels and this will allow surges of HGH production before feedback shuts off the production again.

To emphasize once more, this is an extremely simplified model. There are a great many interactions involved in HGH physiology. The pituitary is something of a master gland which affects many other glands in the endocrine system, and HGH is something of a "master hormone". As such it affects the levels of many other hormones in the body. Notwithstanding these other interactions, the pituitary's principal mode of regulation, vis a vis HGH release, is by the hypothalamus, as described.

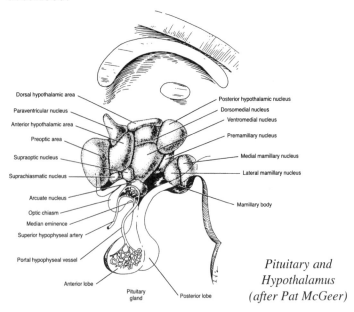

Dorsal hypothalamic area
Paraventricular nucleus
Anterior hypothalamic area
Preoptic area
Supraoptic nucleus
Suprachiasmatic nucleus
Arcuate nucleus
Optic chiasm
Median eminence
Superior hypophyseal artery
Portal hypophyseal vessel
Anterior lobe
Pituitary gland
Posterior lobe

Posterior hypothalamic nucleus
Dorsomedial nucleus
Ventromedial nucleus
Premamillary nucleus
Medial mamillary nucleus
Lateral mamillary nucleus
Mamillary body

Pituitary and Hypothalamus (after Pat McGeer)

If, with all the abbreviations used here, we seem to be thickening an alphabet soup already rich in letters, we might regard the two hormones from the hypothalamus that govern the HGH release from the pituitary merely as Stop and Go. In fact, we might look at the bloodstream as being a large parking lot with a certain number of cars in it, with the cars being molecules of HGH. The hypothalamus would be represented by a counter that kept track of the number of cars (HGH) in the lot, and that also controlled the entrance to the lot with a Stop and a Go sign. As cars (HGH) left the lot at an exit some distance away, thereby making room for more cars (HGH) in the lot, the counter (hypothalamus) would detect this and would flash a Go sign at the entrance. When there were sufficient cars in the lot the counter (hypothalamus) would flash a Stop sign at the entrance. The main point is that the release of HGH by the pituitary is regulated by the hypothalamus as part of a more complex loop.

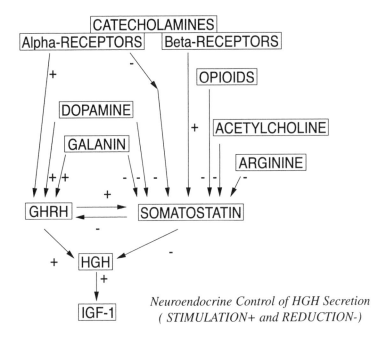

Neuroendocrine Control of HGH Secretion
(STIMULATION+ and REDUCTION-)

The part of the picture that interests us most, however, has to do with the effect of HGH on the rest of the body. Initially, this principally involves the liver. As large volumes of blood are pumped through the liver via the hepatic portal system, the HGH in the blood acts on the liver (amongst other tissues) to stimulate the production of a hormone called Insulin-like Growth Factor-1 (IGF-1) which consists of 70 amino acids, and Insulin-like Growth Factor-2 (IGF-2) which consists of 67 amino acids. It is through IGF-1 that HGH does most of its work.

As the molecules of IGF-1 are carried by binding proteins from the liver to other parts of the body, they attach onto the walls of cells that make up the various organs. From this point on, just how HGH works its magic (in the form of its successor, IGF-1) is not known with absolute certainty. What is known is that IGF-1 with binding protein attaches to cell membrane receptors and stimulates cell differentiation and division, conferring positive effects on cartilage, blood cells, ovarian hormone production, muscle growth and lens differentiation. As well, IGF-1 signals a rejuvenation and restoration in all cells of the body.

Some of the latest research in this area is currently being conducted by Grace Wong of Genentech, where recombinant HGH was first synthesized. Wong theorizes that HGH (in the form of IGF-1) works by intervening in a causal chain in the following way - and here we come back once more to those nasty free radicals.

As our cells produce energy, one of the by-products consists of oxygen based free radicals. In our cells these free radicals in turn activate destructive enzymes called proteases, which attack and damage the protein in our

cells. And when enough damage occurs, the cell dies.
Certain anti-oxidants such as vitamins E and C are able to
nullify some of the action of these free radicals which
stimulate the destructive protease activity. But HGH
works at the problem closer to its source.

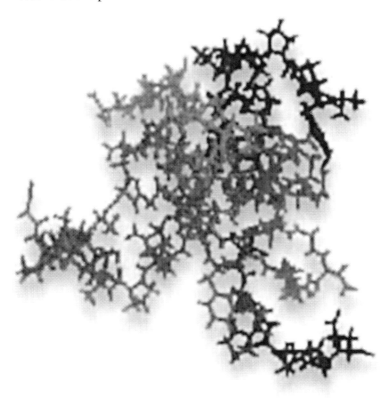

IGF-1 molecule, the hormone we measure to determine HGH activity.

Current research indicates that HGH activates an
innate defense mechanism in the cell which brings forth
substances called protease inhibitors. These protease
inhibitors, as their name suggests, interfere with the
destructive activity of proteases. And these protease
inhibitors are able to do this even when free radicals are
present and "egging" the proteases on.

By way of analogy you might picture this in terms of the automobile. We need the automobile (cellular energy production) and yet the by-product that it gives off, its exhaust (free radicals), is harmful for us to breathe in as we drive along. If we had air filters in our cars that screened out some of the exhaust fumes, that would be somewhat akin to the action of anti-oxidants, which are able to neutralize some of the free radicals and thereby reduce their capacity to activate the destructive proteases.

On the other hand, if we were wearing a mask in the car which was hooked up to an air tank, we would be spared so much more of the harmful effects of the exhaust, even when the exhaust was all around us. And this effect is much like that of HGH in the protease scenario. The HGH, by eliciting the action of protease inhibitors, deters the proteases from going into their destructive action, even when free radicals are present and bidding them (biochemically) to do so.

This is the theory so far, but further experiment is likely to confirm much of it rather than contradict it. By way of partial corroboration, protease inhibitors such as saquinavir and ritonavir are presently being used in the treatment of AIDS patients. Early results so far indicate that they are helping to reduce the levels of the virus in patients to almost undetectable levels.

Wong also theorizes that HGH may be affecting a cell's tendency toward aging by way of countering apoptosis, which is the programmed death of a cell. (As a mnemonic, or memory aid, you might think of apoptosis as the programmed tendency of a cell to eventually die, or "pop off".)

Experiments have demonstrated that when proteases associated with apoptosis are introduced into brain cells, the brain cells die. When these cells are induced to make protease inhibitors, however, the cells survive. Thus, by causing a cell to make protease inhibitors, HGH may well be causing it to stave off "popping off".

To emphasize once more, much that comprises the explanations of how HGH works is still at the theoretical stage, with experimental work presently ongoing. But much of this work is expected to corroborate present theory. What is virtually beyond theory at present is that HGH has shown that it can, to a very considerable extent, counter and halt the aging process. It will be left to the future to explain in detail exactly how it works its wonders. For now, it is enough to know that it does.

Increasing HGH Levels

By the time we reach the age of 25, the pituitary has already begun to release less HGH into the bloodstream. By age 40 our HGH levels are only about 40% of what they were in our prime, around age 20. Since the evidence strongly indicates that these lower levels of HGH play an integral part of the aging process, and that elevating these levels of HGH back to where they were in our younger years can offset the effects of aging, the trick is to do that - to raise the levels of HGH.

Many studies that we have already described - most notably those of Dr. Chein and Dr. Terry at Palm Springs - have shown that injections of HGH do that very effectively. However, this method of treatment has a number of drawbacks. For one thing, injections are very expensive, costing anywhere from hundreds of dollars to a few thousand dollars per month, depending on the individual's requirement. Also, the injections are generally carried out in a clinical or hospital setting, by medical personnel, and require considerable testing and monitoring to keep the proper dosages on track so as to avoid side effects. This is necessary because, when HGH is delivered to the bloodstream by injection, the feedback loop that keeps the HGH levels in the normal range will end up being bypassed, and it is largely when the levels of HGH are raised artificially high that problems tend to occur.

The reason HGH cannot be taken orally as a pill or capsule is that HGH is a large protein. Inside the stomach and intestines we produce enzymes that break HGH down into its component amino acids, just as they would do with a nice steak or bowl of cottage cheese, or any other foodstuff rich in protein.

Also, because of the large size of the HGH molecule, it cannot be absorbed through the skin. Some preparations of HGH have been produced for absorption into the bloodstream through vessels under the tongue, but this method of delivery also has drawbacks, conferring results that are unreliable. Difficulties have to do not only with absorbtion but also with dosage - it is difficult to determine how well HGH will be absorbed in each person and at different times of the day. As a consequence, serum levels can fluctuate beyond what is desirable, again with unwanted side effects. Because HGH is such a large molecule (191 amino acids), it is poorly absorbed by any route except injection, as is the case for Insulin (consisting of 51 amino acids). But where diabetics have the advantage of cheap and convenient blood sugar measurements with a personal glucometer, Growth Hormone Deficient adults (GHD's) have no cheap method yet of watching their IGF-1 levels. However, there is work being done at present to perfect easy saliva testing, which could then be carried out via mail order, or perhaps even with home test kits.

Minimalism

Some years back there was a movement that came to the fore in the art world. It went by the name of Minimalism, and its principal tenet was "Less is More".

Essentially, the movement sought to produce and promote a simplicity in art, to have artworks that were lean and uncluttered. In a word, to produce art that was "Minimal".

Taken to its extremes, perhaps the ultimate offerings from a minimalist's hand - things like an empty canvas or an untouched block of marble - might be things that many would not consider as being art at all; might in fact be things that some would regard with a jaundiced eye, and perhaps even bristle at. One painting of this sort was bought by the Federal Government of Canada during that period, for a large sum of money, and it outraged a good many Canadians.

The painting consisted of three vertical blocks of color that filled a huge canvas, and that was it. The reason for the outrage, aside from the expenditure of taxpayers' money, was that many citizens felt that this painting was too simple, too minimalist to even qualify as art. That it served no purpose.

And yet the Minimalist movement did have a valid point. Paintings, and other artworks, do not always have to be filled with detail and complexity. There is a place for a simple, well done sketch, or a clean, open Chinese ink drawing. Art does not always have to be bigger, fuller, more. There is a place for less. The trick is to get it right.

So too for HGH levels that are artificially altered in the body. Although the desired effect is to raise the depressed levels of HGH above some minimal, inadequate standard, it is not the desired effect to bring about levels that are too high, and that bring on unwanted side effects. Here too, the trick is to get it right.

And this brings us to secretogogues.

Secretogogues

A secretogogue is a substance, chemical, or nutrient which will by its nature encourage a gland to release a hormone. The consequences of achieving this with HGH, of course, are raised levels of HGH in the body.

As we go into middle age and beyond, the pituitary does not stop producing HGH, it just releases less of it into the bloodstream. A particular style of secretogogue can trigger the release of HGH, and in this way is able to bring about higher HGH levels than were occurring previously.

What this means is that, for a forty year old, whose HGH levels have been on the decrease for about twenty years, a secretogogue can raise the concentration of HGH in the bloodstream to a more youthful level. In turn, this affords the possibility of halting much of the aging process, and possibly even reversing some of it.

Because secretogogues bring about the release of HGH from the body's own pituitary, at the body's own rate, the levels of HGH remain subject to governance by the hypothalamus and its feedback loop. Consequently, there is little or no possibility of artificially raising the serum levels of HGH to anything above normal, and consequently again, there is little or no possibility of bringing on serious side effects.

Another advantage to using secretogogues to achieve elevated HGH levels is that the cost of secretogogues is a fraction of that of injections. Also, there are no needles involved, and secretogogues can be taken at home without a medical presence on hand. Finally, because secretogogues are so safe, there is little monitoring required. In short, secretogogues are presently the safest, handiest and most cost effective means of elevating HGH levels in the body.

Secretogogue Agents

Amino Acids

There are a number of substances or agents that act as secretogogues. Some of the most effective and most commonly used are amino acids. Amino acids, we will recall, are the building blocks of protein. Of the twenty-one amino acids needed as part of our physiological requirements, nine of them our bodies cannot make on their own, and must have supplied through diet.

The early, ground-breaking work in the field of oral HGH secretogogues was done by Doctors Isadori, Lo Monoco, and Cappa in 1981 at the University of Rome. In the 1990's, because of both their effectiveness and convenient mode of delivery, secretogogues have undergone a flurry of interest and activity. Numerous studies are ongoing and in the months and years to come, there will be a flood of detailed data concerning them. Recently, writing about amino acids in their role as secretogogues, Dr. Chein, in his new book **"Age Reversal: From Hormones to Telomeres"** has stated, "Researchers have isolated specific amino acids that appear to simulate the release of HGH of the pituitary. By taking supplemental amino acids, you can raise your serum levels...."

Many of the amino acids that serve as HGH releasers have a synergistic effect when used in combination. Preparations of secretogogues that contain a number of amino acids are frequently referred to as amino acid stacks, the term "stack" having been borrowed from the weightlifting community, where it was used to signify a number of preparations used in conjunction with one another. The recent ability to produce crystalline free-form amino acids at relatively low cost, has brought about a revolution in secretogogue technology.

For the list of amino acids that follows, studies have shown some of them to exhibit their own particular beneficial effects, in addition to their effects as HGH releasers. Many marketed HGH releasers are ineffective. **To be effective HGH releasers, specific combinations and amounts of amino acid salts are required.**

Arginine. No doubt the amino acid most commonly used as a secretogogue is arginine. The study by Doctor Isadori and colleagues in Rome showed that as an HGH releaser, Arginine with Lysine even outperformed L-dopa. Arginine has also been shown to increase the body's production of NO (nitric oxide), which allows for penile erections. In addition, its performance as a secretogogue can be enhanced still further when taken in conjunction with other specific amino acid salts.

Lysine. Besides acting on its own in the body by stimulating the secretion of thymic hormone, and by augmenting the body in its use of IGF-1, lysine also provides a synergistic effect when used in conjunction with arginine. Taken together, lysine and arginine make up one of the most commonly used combinations in secretogogue preparations.

Ornithine. Frequently paired with arginine as well, is the amino acid, ornithine. Given that arginine is a biochemical precursor to ornithine, it is not surprising that besides having a synergistic effect with arginine, on its own it also provides some of the same benefits conferred by arginine. In a study by Dirk Pearson and

Sandy Shaw, it was found that taking 5 to 10 grams of this non-essential amino acid on an empty stomach at bedtime appeared to cause HGH secretion to double, although the effects of long term ingestion of such a large amount of this one amino acid are unknown. Ornithine has also been shown to bolster the immune system, aid in liver regeneration, and effect ammonia detoxification.   Ornithine is also found in high concentrations in the skin and connective tissue, suggesting that it may well be useful in maintaining and repairing these tissues. As well, ornithine serves as a precursor of the amino acids citrulline, proline, and glutamic acid.

Glutamine.   Instrumental on its own in raising the levels of HGH, Glutamine is also an integral component of the brain's biochemistry, particularly as to its being converted to glutamic acid. It has also been shown to have a strong effect on the expansion and firmness of muscle.

Leucine. This essential amino acid, branch-chained like valine and isoleucine, makes up about a third of muscle protein. So besides serving as a secretogogue, studies have shown leucine to minimize the loss of muscle mass in patients recovering from surgery or severe trauma.

Glycine.   While glycine also serves as a secretogogue, it is most commonly used in conjunction with arginine and ornithine in raising HGH levels.

Valine.   This is another branched-chain amino acid abundant in muscle tissue. It is a necessary substrate for two other amino acids, glutamine and alanine, which are released in large quantities during intense exercise. Since, like other branched-chain secretogogues, valine is used up by the muscles, it spares other amino acids from being catabolized. Besides having shown itself to be an HGH releaser, it also promotes increased muscle mass and strength, which in turn also helps to offset the aging process.

Carnitine. In addition to functioning as a secretogogue, carnitine also helps promote weight loss. It does this by assisting in transporting long fatty acid chains to muscle tissue, where it can be metabolized.

Tryptophan. This amino acid is a neurotransmitter precursor. It induces a calming effect, so is effective in treating anxiety and stress. Besides acting directly to induce HGH release from the pituitary, it also assists in this by means of its secondary effect of countering insomnia. Since one of the largest pulses of HGH release from the pituitary occurs in early sleep, by acting as a soporific, tryptophan conduces to this end by effecting this valuable early sleep.

Tyrosine. Tyrosine is a biochemical precursor to the neurotransmitter, dopamine. As such it affects HGH levels indirectly. That is, if a reserve of tyrosine is available, dopamine levels can be kept higher; and dopamine, amongst other things, acts as an HGH releaser. Tyrosine also produces a stimulating effect and blocks the calming and soporific effects of tryptophan. It also improves nerve transmission from the brain to the muscles, stimulating more motor units and conferring higher strength levels. There is some attenuation of its effects and therefore it should not be used on a regular, ongoing basis.

Gamma Amino butyric Acid (GABA). GABA acts as an effective HGH releaser and confers a pleasant, relaxing, calming effect, somewhat in the manner of tryptophan.

Drugs

The one drug we will look at here that acts as an HGH releaser is a drug we just touched upon above, L-dopa. Amongst its other properties, L-dopa is an excellent secretogogue.   Since it is an amino acid precursor to several neurotransmitters that control pituitary function, it is thereby a very effective secretogogue.

A study conducted in 1982 involved the treatment of rats with L-dopa. The results of this study were that the rats showed raised levels of serum and pituitary levels of GH. In addition, the older rats regained levels of GH that were in line with those exhibited by young rats.

Also, it has been shown that IGF-1 levels do not decrease after years of treatment with L-dopa for Parkinson's disease or for Nocturnal Leg Cramps.

Research data on L-dopa has shown that it is a powerful drug, and as such, remains available only by prescription.

HGH Enhancement

Besides raising HGH levels directly by injection, or by the use of secretogogues, there are still other ways to enhance HGH levels in the body. And although they may not demonstrate as dramatic an effect as shown by injections or secretogogues, these methods are capable of bringing about increased levels of HGH. Where these enhancers are used in conjunction with each other, *and most particularly with the use of secretogogues*, you have the recipe for attaining excellent HGH levels, without the use of injections.

Diet

Since most of the secretogogues consist of amino acids, which are the building blocks of protein, we would do well to include sufficient quantities of complete proteins in our diet. Foodstuffs like meat, poultry, fish, tofu, and cottage cheese are all excellent sources of protein and have been promoted lately with diets like *The Zone, Protein Power* and *Dr. Atkins Diet*

Besides the amino acids already mentioned, there are some B vitamins that have also demonstrated the capacity to act as HGH releasers. These include vitamin B6 and niacin.

You Are What You Eat. This expression was making the rounds some years back, and there is a great deal of truth in it. If we do not embrace a good, all-round diet, our health in general suffers, and this will reflect itself in many ways, including our manufacture and output of HGH. Therefore, in addition to taking secretogogues and ensuring an intake rich in protein, one would be wise to effect a diet that considered all aspects of nutrition, about which more will be said later.

You Are As Much As You Eat. This statement might hold another bit of "food for thought". That is, the more we eat - over and above an optimal limit - the more we will pack on as fat. Even if it is food that is good for us. And these extra pounds of fat will, especially when occurring in abundance, have a deleterious effect on our health. In addition to the expected hazards to our health (increased risk of heart attack, diabetes, etc.), one study showed that fat, along with age, correlated significantly with reduced levels of HGH in the body. To put it another way, the study indicated that the levels of HGH tended to be affected by these two factors (age and obesity), so that lower levels of HGH tended to be found in older subjects of similar weight groups, as well as in overweight subjects of similar age groups.

In view of this finding, for people who are overweight, cutting down on the food intake will provide not only the normal, expected benefits, but will also confer the bonus of promoting higher HGH levels in the body. As well, there is a happy cyclical interaction at work here: the more fat that is lost, the higher the HGH levels a person can expect to have; and the higher the HGH levels a person has, the greater the tendency to drop the fat.

Fasting

You Are What You Don't Eat. When thought of in terms of fasting, this is another thought that we might keep in mind when striving for higher HGH levels. That is because fasting has also been shown to increase the levels of HGH in the body.

As a species, we have been subject to fasting throughout most of our history. Prior to the invention of agriculture, obtaining food was a chancy and spotty business. Even after the establishment of agriculture, many people have been subject to bouts of fasting, or at least to periods of low caloric intake. As well, most of the major religions have traditionally called for periods of fasting during particular periods on their religious calendars. Oddly, unless carried to extremes, rather than being harmed by fasting, human beings seem to benefit from fasting. Perhaps being positively impacted by fasting is something of a defence mechanism that has come about because we have been subjected to fasting over the millennia.

The current popular explanation for the perceived beneficial effects of fasting is that fasting allows the digestive system a chance to rest, to eliminate foreign substances, and that fasting allows the body to cleanse itself of metabolic impurities.

Just how fasting tends to promote higher HGH levels is, up to this point, not well understood. Perhaps the theorizing that Jens Sandahl Christiansen has done with regard to the interaction and effect of blood glucose levels, insulin levels, and HGH levels - as they fluctuate after a meal - will offer some clues. For these three factors do appear to be interacting, however directly or indirectly, in some kind of physiological dance.

Initially after eating a meal, blood glucose levels rise, as do the levels of insulin, which rise sharply. The insulin promotes the storage of excess carbohydrate and fat. During this phase the levels of HGH change little and remain low.

Over the next two hours the blood glucose and the insulin levels begin to decline, while those of HGH begin to rise slowly. At this stage HGH is promoting the buildup of muscle, its function enhanced by the presence of insulin.

In the last stage, four hours after eating, the blood glucose levels remain low, the insulin levels hit their lowest point, but in contrast, the levels of HGH reach and remain at their highest point. During this phase it is mainly HGH alone that functions in promoting the burning of fat stores in the body. Finally, after six hours, the HGH levels begin to drop as well.

Given Christiansen's explanation of what is occurring with respect to the levels of these three substances, one might be tempted to speculate just a little as to how this might offer an explanation concerning the raised HGH levels that occur during fasting. Could it be that since there is no food coming into the digestive system, the blood glucose levels then remain low, and as a consequence, so do the insulin levels? Perhaps, with the body still needing energy for its day to day activities, and if the function of HGH in this context is in facilitating the burning of fat stores in the body, then that function would require that HGH continue to be present at high levels. Which is exactly where the levels of HGH are found to be during fasting.

On the other hand, perhaps other explanations will be found that demonstrate the situation to be otherwise.

Exercise

We have all seen the benefits of exercise (if not in the mirror, then on others): muscles rippling and well defined; contours of marble; skin glowing and smooth; a bounce in the step - all indicators of a strength and endurance within. But there is yet another benefit of exercise, a benefit more subtle than the others, and it too is found within: higher HGH levels.

It should not come as a complete surprise that this is so. We know that exercise is good for us, that it can help keep us trim, firm, and slow down the aging process. And we know that this is also the case for HGH, although at a higher degree of efficacy. So it should not be surprising to see that exercise has been shown to elevate the levels of HGH in the body. In fact, it would actually seem quite plausible that the increased levels of HGH generated by heavy exercise is in part, at least, the mechanism by which the anti-aging results are ultimately obtained.

And here again we see HGH involved in a cyclical relationship: exercise (muscle mass working) promotes raised HGH levels; raised HGH levels contribute to the formation of new muscle mass; which can do even more exercise, and so on.

To be precise, the kind of exercise that is most conducive to raised HGH levels is that of a non-aerobic, strength producing nature. Exercises with weights, for example, that are done for strength and not endurance, where the body is pushed to its limit within a few repetitions - these are the kinds of exercises that raise the levels of HGH. Similarly, a hard driving game of squash or tennis is more efficacious in raising HGH levels than is a more leisurely game over a longer period of time.

A study that supports this very well, involved a number of women divided into three groups; the first group would run a set distance of about 40 miles in a week, doing a third of this distance on three different days, running it at their flat out limit. The second group would cover the same distance, but it was spread out over six days, and was run at a more moderate pace. The third group was a control group and did not run at all.

Somewhat surprisingly, only the first group showed strong increases in their HGH bursts or pulse levels. Undoubtedly, the second group would have benefitted by strengthening the cardiovascular system, as well as by gains in muscle tone and by burning off calories. But they did not show the solid HGH gains made by the first group that ran harder and faster.

Of course, as was expected, the control group showed no change in HGH levels.

Other studies have also come up with similar results. The upshot is, to raise the levels of HGH significantly by means of exercise, strenuous exercise works best.

It is possible that lower body exercises are more effective that upper body workouts for raising HGH levels. If so, that may simply reflect the fact that the quadriceps and other leg muscles are amongst the largest in the body, and for that reason should be more effective in raising HGH levels.

An added benefit to extended, strenuous exercise, is the mild feeling of euphoria that often comes with it, brought on by elevated levels of beta endorphins in the brain. Additionally, these raised levels of endorphins have been shown to promote the secretion of HGH. To what extent this represents the mechanism by which exercise raises the levels of HGH is unknown. In fact, it is little understood at all just why exercise brings about raised levels of HGH. Undoubtedly, this is just one more area currently being researched in this interesting and exciting field.

Sleep

Sleep is particularly important in enhancing the levels of HGH. We have already seen that the strongest bursts or pulses of HGH occur about one or two hours after we first fall asleep at night, particularly in men. Obviously, then, if we get to bed late, or at irregular hours, and if our sleep is interrupted and broken with shift work or emotional upset, we will likely interfere with these pulses. However, if we choose a secretogogue with an amino acid stack containing one of them that is conducive to drowsiness, this will help us to get to sleep so that we may attain these high HGH pulses. Since HGH has been found to improve our sleep, once again we arrive at a cyclical situation. Raised HGH levels by use of secretogogues help us to sleep better; sleeping better helps the pituitary release more optimal pulses of HGH.

With more and more evidence accruing, all attesting to the importance of sleep to our health, this also accentuates the need for optimal HGH levels. Men, in particular, are susceptible to lowered HGH levels from poor sleep habits, because men require the deep sleep more than do women to effect the large burst of HGH release that takes place an hour or so after falling asleep. Women are less dependent on the large burst of HGH that takes place in the early period of deep sleep, because they also have a propensity to release HGH in smaller bursts throughout the day. Given that, traditionally, more men have worked night shifts and swing shifts, it could be that this is a relevant factor in the shorter life span men have compared to women. Losing REM sleep may cause psychological problems, but a lack of deep sleep for men may actually be shortening their lives.

Certainly, work with amino acid secretogogues has shown that women may take their amino acids through the day, but men have much better results (higher IGF-1 levels) if the amino acids are taken before bed.

Studies continue to show us that longevity is maximized with an 8 hour sleep schedule.

Putting it All Together

With all of the studies that have already been completed, and with corroborating data continuing to pour in, there is little doubt left that HGH is the best defense so far against the aging process - the biggest bullet in the armamentarium.

Dr. Chein and Dr. Terry have produced an abundance of data detailing the efficacy and the safety of HGH when proper dosages and schedules are followed.

And now, offering even greater safety and convenience, we have the means to increase our levels of HGH, on our own, at home, by the use of secretogogues. Since secretogogues work by stimulating the pituitary gland to secrete more HGH in our bodies, we do not have to worry about the levels becoming too high. Because HGH is being produced and released by our own bodies, it is subject to our body's feedback loop and control mechanisms.

Given that appropriate exercise, proper diet, and adequate sleep all act as natural HGH releasers, an ideal program suggests that we put it all together. Certainly we can derive wonderful benefits from just the secretogogues alone, and that is the course chosen by some. But since exercise and sleep need not cost anything, and we have to buy food anyway, arguably the "best bang for the buck" would be to combine all of these elements into a program with secretogogues. In such a program, an individual would achieve the increased HGH levels induced by the secretogogues, augmented and enhanced still further by proper exercise, diet, and sleep.

Admittedly, this regime will not allow us to live

forever, but it will almost certainly add many years to our lives, and add life to our years.

There is one last point to be made here, and there is an old joke that may (if only marginally) illustrate it. There were two men out hiking in the woods, when off in the distance they spied a large bear starting into a charge at them. The first guy bends over to tighten his shoelaces, as if in preparation for a run. The second guy says to him, "You don't think you will be able to outrun the bear, do you?" And the first guy says, "I don't have to outrun the bear - all I have to do is outrun you!"

What this joke illustrates for us is that we may sometimes achieve a goal in an indirect or roundabout way.

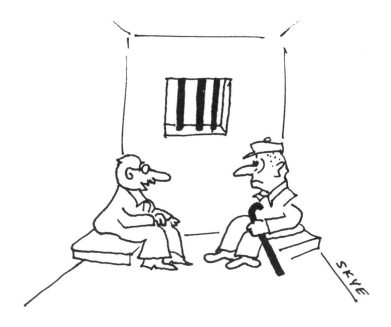

Do you want to continue your longevity program here?

By embarking on a program to increase our levels
of HGH, we know that it is not going to enable us to live
forever. But such a program may take us further along
to where the next discovery may. Or the one after that.
Because at the rate new discoveries are being made
nowadays, who can say?

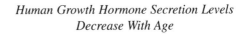

*Human Growth Hormone Secretion Levels
Decrease With Age*

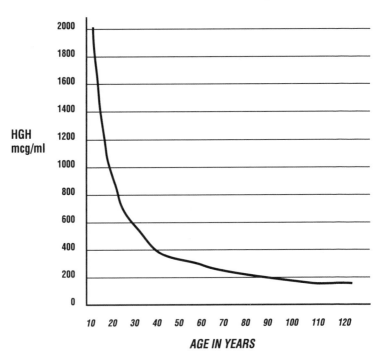

[At a symposium given by Dr. White and Dr.
McLeod, one participant remarked that unless he could
convince his friends to raise their HGH output, then he
may end up with few friends when he is 120 years
young.]

FACTORS THAT AFFECT HUMAN
GROWTH HORMONE SECRETION

INCREASE HGH	DECREASE HGH
PHYSIOLOGICAL	
DEEP SLEEP STRENUOUS EXERCISE STRESS CONDITIONS PROTEIN INGESTION FASTING	HYPERGLYCEMIA FREE FATTY ACIDS
PHARMACOLOGICAL	

INSULIN WITH HYPOGLYCEMIA
POST GLUCAGON
HORMONES:
  HGH RELEASING HORMONE
  VASOPRESSIN, ACTH
  ESTROGENS
  PEPTIDES (hexarelin)
NEUROTRANSMITTERS:
  ALPHA ADRENERGIC AGONISTS
   (clonidine)
  BETA ADRENERGIC ANTAGONISTS
   (inderal and other beta blockers)
  SEROTONIN PRECURSORS
   (also SSRI's like prozac)
  DOPAMINE AGONISTS
   (levodopa, apomorphine, bromocriptine)
  GABA AGONISTS (muscimol)
  MELATONIN
POTASSIUM I.V.
PYROGENS (BACTERIAL TOXINS)
AMINO ACIDS (arginine, lysine, ornithine)
	HORMONES:
	  SOMATOSTATIN
	  HGH
	  PROGESTERONE
	  CORTISOL ETC.
	NEUROTRANSMITTERS:
	  ALPHA A. ANTAGONIST
	   (phentolomine)
	  BETA A. AGONISTS
	   (isoproteronol)
	  SEROTONIN BLOCKERS
	   (methysergide)
	  DOPA ANTAGONISTS
	   (phenothiazines)

DISEASES	
STARVATION AND ANOREXIA NERVOSA CHRONIC RENAL FAILURE ACROMEGALY	OBESITY DWARFISM THYROID DISEASE

Benefits of HGH

So far we have looked at the benefits of HGH sporadically, or in the form of lists and statistics. But to fully appreciate the benefits of HGH we might want to take a closer look, to examine in more detail its effects on our organs and tissues, where HGH actually does its work.

Fat Loss

When the bubonic plague struck Europe centuries back, it struck down over a third of the population. If a plague of that magnitude were upon us today our heads of government would be mobilizing all possible forces to counteract it.

Yet there is a plague of sorts upon us, the plague of obesity. More than a third of all North Americans are overweight or obese. And although this plague does not have people dying in the streets, it does subject them to very serious health risks.

Aesthetic aspects aside, those carrying the extra pounds also carry with them a greater tendency for heart attack, stroke, diabetes, atherosclerosis, and even problems with arthritis.

Yet it's not that those carrying the extra pounds don't care, that they are not doing something about it. There is, in fact, a mighty effort on the part of these people to drop the pounds. As a testament to this effort one need only look at the best seller list - rarely is it without some kind of diet book included. Ditto for TV - endless ads for this diet milkshake, or that weight loss plan. And think back to all the weight loss gizmos and gadgets - if we had a dollar for each one gathering cobwebs in the attics and basements of America, we'd be rich.

It's not as though these attempts at weight loss have been wholly ineffective. Many people have lost weight - for a time. But then they put it all back on again, often with a few extra pounds to boot. So the weight goes on and off, on and off, again and again. The yo-yo effect.

Concerning personal finances there is an old saying: If your outgo exceeds your income, your upkeep will be your downfall. In weight loss the opposite is true: If the incoming calories exceed the outgoing calories, this will be your downfall. Weight loss will not occur.

The incoming calories derive from one source only, from what we consume, from what we eat or drink.

The outgoing calories, on the other hand, the calories we expend, can be looked at as being used up via two different modes. The first mode is the heightened expenditure of calories through exercise. A rodeo rider making eight (staying up on a Brahma bull or a bucking bronco for eight seconds) is using up a lot of energy, a lot of calories with this exercise.

A couch potato, in contrast, uses up fewer calories making eight, unless the "eight" is in reference to "eight hours". Nevertheless, the couch potato does burn up calories just lying there. In fact, even when we are at complete rest we all burn up calories at a lower rate called the basal metabolic rate.

For some people, this basal metabolic rate is higher, and more calories are used up while they are at rest. For others it is lower, and fewer calories are used up while they are at rest. For people in a given age group, these differences in basal metabolic rate can manifest themselves in obvious ways. For instance, those with the lower metabolic rate are the ones that can, seemingly, just walk by a breadbox and put on a pound or two. Those in the other group - the ones with the higher metabolic rate - can swallow an entire bakery and remain lean.

Individual differences aside, there is one major generality that holds for all: as we age, our basal metabolic rate tends to become lower. This means that if a twenty year old and a fifty year old sit watching TV, the fifty year old will ordinarily burn fewer calories.

Which brings us to HGH. One of the most dramatic and pronounced effects of HGH therapy is seen in fat loss. This has been observed from Dr. Rudman's early study right on through studies to the present. Perhaps fat loss appears as the most dramatic effect because it is something that the eye can see so readily.

The reason the term "fat" loss is used instead of "weight" loss, is that where people are not greatly overweight, in treatments with HGH they may not even lose any weight. But it will change places, and it will change in composition. Weight will move from the waist to the arms, legs, the shoulders. It will change from fat to muscle. Through this loss of fat and gain in muscle the body will become reconfigured. Through the effects of raised HGH levels we are returned to our more youthful shapes, our more youthful figures.

Although this loss of fat and gain in muscle mass is readily detected by others, it is the physiological changes within that are important. For they are the changes that cause the outer changes.

The Workings of HGH

The fat cells in our bodies have receptor sites where HGH and IGF-1 may bind to the cell. Once attached, HGH and IGF-1 set up a series of reactions in the cell's biochemistry, the end result of which is the breakdown in fat. You might look at HGH as the crank that came with the old Model T Ford. The crank, when put in place to where it hooked up to the motor, could be turned quickly, causing the engine to turn over and start, burning fuel in the cylinders to provide energy and motive power to the car.

So too, when HGH attaches to a fat cell: it cranks the cell into starting the reactions which bring about the breakdown of fat, a process called lypolysis. When the fat is broken down in the body it may then serve as fuel to be burned by the body, thereby providing energy and motive power.

Another explanation concerning a different operation of HGH was put forth by Dr. Rudman and colleagues. This hypothesis looked at HGH as something of an insulin "blocker" in fat cell production. While insulin acts to promote lypogenesis (creation of fat in fat cells), Rudman theorizes that HGH promotes lypolysis, the destruction of fat in fat cells. In this model, insulin works on a cell so as to promote the entry of amino acids, glucose, and fats. In opposition to this, HGH works to block insulin in this function, keeping the fat cells from growing larger.

Diabetes Type 2 is becoming endemic in North America, with estimates of up to 10% of the population affected. Its rise in the 30-40 age group coincides with the obesity and poor dietary habits seen in America today.

Given these figures, the importance of HGH as an agent in bringing about fat loss is once again underscored. And no matter how the details of the physiology of HGH come to be understood ultimately, the conclusion that HGH does bring about fat loss is uncontested.

The Pear and the Apple

There are two main body shapes that tend to occur in people who are overweight. One is the pear shape, where much of the fat accumulates around the hips and buttocks. Although far from benign, fat located in these areas tends to bring on fewer health problems than does fat that occurs in the second, or apple shape.

The apple shape is the one where the fat accumulates around the middle: gut fat. This accumulation of fat gives the torso of the overweight person the roundedness of an apple - a sort of roly-poly Tweedledee or Tweedledum kind of shape. You might consider this fat as dumb fat, or Tweedledumb fat, since it is this fat, bulging out around the waist, that most tends to correlate with health problems. It is the Tweedledumb fat that tends most to increase the odds for heart disease and diabetes.

Another negative impact of this Tweedledumb fat is that it also tends to correlate with lower levels of HGH.

HGH vs Tweedledumb

As doctors of the baby boomer athletes, we constantly hear of the difficulty our patients have trying to lose the spare tire. Exercise seldom cancels out this fat storage problem in the middle years.

There have been many studies which point up the effectiveness of HGH in bringing about the necessary fat loss. We have already seen some of the results obtained in patients by Dr. Chein and Dr. Terry at Palm Springs.

As for that central fat around the waist - the Tweedledumb fat - HGH is particularly effective in bringing about its reduction and loss. In one study by Dr. Bengt-Ake Bengtssön at Sahlgrenska Hospital in Sweden, adults deficient in HGH were treated with this hormone for six months. Over this period, the patients in this study lost 20 % of their body fat. Even more encouraging were the numbers for fat loss around the mid-section, the Tweedledumb fat. Here, 30% of the fat was lost.

It is especially difficult for older people to shed Tweedledumb fat, and more difficult still to lose fat associated with this Tweedledumb fat that builds up internally, in the body cavity around various organs. You can do arm exercises, leg exercises, even sit-ups to work off the outer fat. But there is little by way of exercise that readily works off these central, internal fat deposits. And yet here, too, HGH has shown itself to be amazingly effective.

In another study at Sahlgrenska, Gudmundar Johannson, Bengt-Ake Bengtssön, and colleagues used low dose injections on healthy older men over a period of nine months. The results were impressive: an average loss of 9.2% of total body fat; a 6.1% loss of abdominal fat; and a marvellous 18.1% of internal, central body fat. All without additional diet or exercise!

These treatments had been conducted as a double

blind study with one group serving as a control group. By the end of the study, the control group had actually put on more fat.

Those in the study receiving the HGH treatments, besides losing impressive amounts of fat, also showed an improved cholesterol profile, a lower level of blood triglycerides, lower blood pressure, and an improved glucose metabolism.

In a study conducted by Belgian physician, Thierry Hertoghe, further impressive results were obtained. This study involved making careful and detailed body measurements at the start. Then, over a two month period, HGH and other hormones that had been in decline, were administered. Hertoghe found a 20 to 30 percent shrinkage in the love handles on patients, as well as shrinkage in the abdomen, and even in the underside of the thigh. Indicative of this shrinkage of body fat in general, Hertoghe found that the belly buttons of these patients moved up by more than an inch by the end of the study. More striking yet, Hertoghe is of the opinion that the loose skin hanging from the upper arms on some women are signs of lower HGH levels, and that as levels of HGH are restored, so too this flappy skin will improve and tighten up. At last, something that appears to work on those unsightly triceps wattles.

Priming the Pump

We have seen that obesity tends to bring on lowered levels of HGH. This provokes an intriguing thought: Would it be possible, in people who are obese, to induce a restored level of HGH?

A research group in Santiago, Spain, headed up by

Fernando Cordido, set up an experiment to answer just that question. They used a combination of Growth Hormone Releasing Hormone (GHRH) with a new HGH releasing drug called GHRP 6. Treating patients who were more than 130 % over their ideal weight, Cordido found that the two substances produced a powerful synergistic effect. The patients exhibited huge releases of HGH. Cordido had demonstrated "...that the blunted GH secretion in obesity is a functional and potentially reversible state."

It is possible to prime the pump!

Where this result will lead upon further experimentation is anybody's guess. But it does underscore once more that in the field of anti-aging, the possibilities appear unbounded.

HGH: Muscle Mass Maker

On the flip side of the ability of HGH to bring about fat loss, is its ability to bring about gains in muscle mass. Again, there has been study after study that has confirmed this result.

The way HGH helps the body build muscle is in its ability to promote reactions that generate new protein, new cells. It does this while operating in the guise of its successor, IGF-1. As IGF-1, it stimulates the uptake of amino acids, which are the building blocks of protein. This, in turn, increases the synthesis of DNA, RNA, proteins, and extracellular proteins, all of which engenders an increase in both cell size and the rate of cell division.

HGH also promotes the conserving of nitrogen in

the body. Since nitrogen is an essential element in amino acids, and therefore in muscle, this helps keep its stock from being diminished or depleted. In the 2000 Olympics, testing of IGF-1 levels was a hot issue due to the unfair advantage athletes have with the higher levels. Most athletes now use amino acid stacks to improve their performance - safely.

Increased Mobility, Decreased Debility

The action of HGH in promoting gains in lean body mass has been demonstrated for people in various categories: weight-lifters, body builders; those who were overweight, those wasting away; those in their younger years (with pituitary deficiencies), those in their declining years. Although HGH has been shown to benefit all, it especially shows great promise for seniors.

HGH has demonstrated not only the ability to promote gains in muscle mass for the elderly, but it also promotes gains in bone mass, bone density. Stronger bones and stronger muscles in those of advancing years means there will be increased mobility, decreased debility. There will be fewer falls, fewer broken bones, especially broken hips. For those who are getting along in years, it will mean that they need not be stuck in a chair for endless hours. And although they may not be able to do the high jump, they will be able to perform many everyday tasks, like going for walks, or preparing meals. For the elderly, HGH will not only mean greater strength, it will mean freedom.

Tip of the Iceberg

Because fat is an outward sign of health risks within,

it is a bit like the tip of an iceberg. In the case of an iceberg, it is not the visible part above water the that causes problems, but rather that which lies below the water, unseen, that can do us harm. So too it is with fat. It is not the visible fat on the outside that actually does us harm, but rather, it is the inner conditions indicated by the fat that cause the problems.

Conditions such as high levels of cholesterol, high triglycerides, high blood pressure, impaired glucose metabolism - these unseen conditions in our physiology are what lead to heart attack, stroke, and diabetes. And it is at this unseen level that HGH does its work. HGH promotes the normalizing of our physiology. It brings about the physiology that we had operating in us a decade or two earlier, which then brings about the body that we had a decade or two earlier. That is how HGH achieves its results.

Given how HGH is able to make us lean and make us muscled, in years to come we may well come to look upon HGH as the modern sculptor, working on the human form.

Appearance

One point that we did not examine while looking at fat loss was appearance. Although our appearance may not directly affect our physical health, it does have an impact indirectly, through our psychological state. We all want to look our best, and when we do not, our self-esteem suffers, often affecting our physical health more than we might guess. Because ultimately, the mind and body are one entity.

Moreover, although emphasis on appearance may strike some as superficial, like it or not, we live in a world where appearances count. And they count big. There are the old bromides that may suggest otherwise "You can't judge a book by its cover." "Clothes don't make the man." but in the world of today, appearance is important.

Perhaps it has to do with the pace of everyday life. We meet dozens of people a day, some for only a moment or two. Often during these moments it is necessary that we make an instantaneous judgment about a person. For instance, if someone in a department store is trying to sell us something, one of the most influencing factors is the salesperson's demeanor and appearance. So appearance is important. And one of the most important features of our appearance is our face.

A New Wrinkle on Wrinkles

To underscore the importance of our facial appearance, all we have to do is look at the attention being paid to the face nowadays - especially by those who are just now leaving behind the bloom of youth.

No doubt, people have always sought to keep the face young. Most potions and home remedies of the past, however, were largely ineffectual. But in the last few decades there has been a strong surge in the output of new products breaking onto the scene: mud packs, moisturizers, facial peels, and the like. For the most part they had two things in common - they were of limited efficacy, and they all worked (where they worked at all) from the outside in.

One recent technique that especially accentuates the importance of appearance involved people having their own fat sucked out of one part of the body, and having it then injected into various parts of the face. The intent was to offset the wrinkles there by filling them in and pressing them out with the injected fat.

Most often, fat was taken from the buttocks because it was usually plentiful there, and it was easy to get at. The reason a person's own fat was used was so that there would be no problems with rejection. No doubt, more than one wag has quipped about the possibility of rejection for other than genetic reasons; namely, that perhaps areas of the face, particularly around the lips, might be inclined to reject material from the buttocks on aesthetic grounds!

Most of the recent skin treatments, however, have been of the standard sort that are rubbed onto the surface of the skin. Some of these topical applications - creams, lotions, etc. - show some ability in restoring the skin, but their effects are usually limited, showing up only on the outermost layer of the skin, at best removing only very fine lines. HGH, in contrast, works on the inner physiology to effect its repairs.

We might compare the two processes to two different methods of repairing a leaky roof on a house. One is to slap some tar paper over the leaky area, and the problem is solved. Sort of. Another way is to go to the heart of the matter, and start by reinforcing any underlying beams and struts that may have begun to rot from the water; then replace weakened boards or plywood under the worn shingles; and finally, replace the worn shingles themselves. Which of the two repair jobs would you prefer?

HGH works along the lines of the second method. It works on the fundamentals within to effect the desired changes without. For one thing, it extends the number of times a skin cell in the dermal layer may divide.

As these cells get older, they do not function as well as they did formerly. HGH, along with other growth factors, has shown itself to be effective in restoring these cells to a more youthful efficiency in carrying out their normal maintenance work.

HGH promotes the restoration of our physiology to what it had been years earlier. It stimulates an increase in the body's production of protein needed in the formation of collagen and elastin, two of the main substances that make up the skin. As it does in the rest of the body, HGH also promotes increased muscle growth in the face, which, along with the renewed collagen and elastin, rebuilds and reconfigures the substructure under the skin. Like the injections of fat, this renewed substructure presses the skin out, but unlike the fat injections, this is renewed muscle and skin, not fat off the buttocks which will be reabsorbed by the body in time.

As HGH stimulates the body to generate more of

these basic building materials, it begins to fill in the facial fissures, to take up the slack in the sagging skin by renewing it as well. It rebuilds from within, pressing out against the skin, and at the same time the renewed skin is drawn more taut over this new substructure. In a word, it makes the skin smoother.

Other than the surgery involved in face lifts, or injections of fat into parts of the face, all other wrinkle remedies work from the outside in. Only HGH uses the body's own chemistry to reduce or eliminate wrinkles from within.

Obviously, since it has taken years for the wrinkles to materialize, they will not be made to recede overnight. Usually, because it is effecting a rebuilding of our anabolic chemistry, it will take some weeks for the effects to be noticed. But noticed they will be.

At Palm Springs, Dr. Chein and Dr. Terry produced marvelous results. In the study mentioned earlier, the results reported for improved skin texture, thickness, and elasticity were all around the 70% mark (71%, 68%, and 71%, respectively). For the disappearance of wrinkles altogether, the figure was an amazing 51%.

The effects of HGH on the skin are not that unlike the effects of a face lift - except that with a face lift the same old skin is simply cut and tucked over the same old shrinking framework underneath. With HGH therapy, we bring about the rebuilding of the musculature below, and the restoration of the collagen and elastin tissues in the skin itself. By promoting the continued cell division in the dermal layer, it reconstitutes the skin to make it thicker and younger. Once a face lift is completed, the skin and the unremedied substructure underneath - continue on their course of withering and decay. With

HGH therapy, the rebuilding and rejuvenating will continue on into the future.

Fine Wine

We have all seen grapes in their prime at the produce store, smooth skinned and almost bursting with juices. We have also seen them desiccated and wrinkled, in the form of raisins.

Where the aging process has taken us to the point where we might be compared to raisins, HGH will not likely restore us to where we might be compared to a new grape. But it will make improvements. And when therapy is begun early enough, then much of the youthful grape may be recaptured, such that there is a firmness to the flesh and a smoothness to the skin, and the juices are again replenished within. With ongoing treatment, we may then - to drastically mix our metaphors - continue aging like grapes of a fine vintage, that ultimately produce a fine wine.

A Beautiful Truth

> *"Beauty is truth, truth beauty - that is all Ye know on earth, and all ye need to know."*

It has been almost two hundred years since romantic poet, John Keats, wrote those words, yet they are as compelling today as they were when first they flowed from his pen. We live our lives by truth, we live our lives for beauty.

We use truth, our perception of the world around us, to order our lives, to improve our lives. And one of the more important improvements includes making the things around us more beautiful, and as well, making ourselves more beautiful.

To date, HGH is almost certainly the best single therapy for helping us to keep the years at arms length and thereby maintain the beauty of our younger selves. The pre-eminence of HGH stems from the fact that it achieves its effects by prompting the body to recharge and restore itself to the body chemistry of its bygone years. It is by taking our body chemistry back in time, by fleshing out our bodies and our faces to their younger contours, that HGH is able to confer upon us the earlier beauty of our younger years. And in so doing, HGH, itself, becomes a beautiful truth.

Hair

Perhaps a sign of aging that is even more visible than wrinkles, is grey hair. Or hair loss. When we consider the number of hair dyes on the market today, we get something of an idea as to how important our appearance is.

Even more telling is the number of baldness "remedies" that have come down the pike over the decades. Unhappily, except for transplants, none has ever truly done the job. There are as many bald people as ever.

We have seen in the Palm Springs data of Dr. Chein and Dr. Terry that there was some success in the regrowth of hair. But it is in this area that HGH has had some of its spottiest results.

There has not been a great deal of research done

specifically on the effects of HGH and hair regrowth - most have concentrated on more serious aspects of health. Having said that, there is, nevertheless, significant collateral evidence that HGH does have a partial effect in producing hair in areas that were previously balding. The Palm Springs study did, if we recall, show reports of 38% for new hair growth, which is considerably better than most products designed specifically to grow hair.

Other studies, as well as those done at Palm Springs, have had patients and researchers alike remarking on how HGH brought about improved hair growth. And more studies yet reporting improved hair color, sometimes even to where the original hair color had been regained. Also, in many of these patients, the texture and luster of their hair had been restored to how it had been years earlier.

Although much of the data on hair growth is anecdotal, it must be borne in mind that in most of these studies, hair growth was not the reason for the HGH therapy in the first place. Which is why a lot of the information concerning hair growth has not been gathered in a rigorously scientific manner. Other methods for hair growth stimulation with the standard finasteride and minoxidil combinations for male pattern baldness we continue to use with moderate success.

Inside Out

A comedian once observed: "Do you realize that all the hair on the outside of your head was once on the inside of your head?"

The reason the line is funny is because of the bizarre

picture it generates - the skull crammed with all that hair. And yet there is a measure of truth implied by the observation. Hair growth does begin on the inside. Perhaps not in great bushy balls, and perhaps not inside the skull itself. But it does grow out of the follicles that extend down into the inner layers of skin.

Since HGH does exercise a broad effect on our physiology, making it "younger", it would be surprising if it did not improve hair growth, as well as hair color and hair texture. Further, with all the research going on at present, the possibility is far from remote that HGH, working in combination with other therapies, may show even more impressive results in the future.

Inner Organs

While appearance is important, our inner health - the condition of our inner organs - is crucial. We can, if we must, live with aging skin that feels like parchment, or hair that looks and feels more and more like porcupine quills. But organs like the heart, the lungs, or the liver we cannot live without. They are necessary for life. And even having these organs working away inside us is not enough. They must be working well.

When organs like the heart or liver are not working well, we are not working well. And when we are not working well, we are not living well.

There is a certain redundancy built into the body. We have two kidneys, two lungs, three lobes to the liver. This means that if one kidney becomes diseased, we can get by with the other one. Or if any of these organ systems is not working at optimal capacity, we can still get by. But in this circumstance we will find that we are far from living at optimal capacity. We are not living a good life. We are slower, or we live in pain and discomfort, or sometimes we "just don't feel well".

This is particularly the case as our inner organs age. Because these organs do age, along with the rest of us. As in the case of skin tissue, for example, our inner organs undergo a certain amount of programmed cell death, a certain amount of shrinkage, which eventually manifests itself as partial impairment. Because of some of the built-in redundancy, however, we will not notice the effects at first. We begin aging while in our twenties, but we usually don't notice it till later.

Once the impairment of function of any of these organs is more advanced, and the deterioration more pronounced, our lives then become that much more limited. We do continue to live, but not nearly so well. Certainly not with the same breadth and scope we enjoyed previously. We find that we can no longer walk as far, or as fast, or as painlessly. Other activities are fraught with similar limitations. With further malfunction of these inner organs, we may find we can only get by with serious medication, or by keeping an oxygen bottle handy, or by making frequent trips to a clinic or hospital to undergo dialysis. But this is not the way it has to be. Just as HGH has been shown to slow or reverse the aging process in other parts of the body, so too it is for our inner organs.

Because HGH works on our fundamental physiology, by this means it also works to improve the health of our inner organs. Because HGH stimulates the emergence of a more youthful body chemistry within us, it is thereby able to make our vital organs more youthful as well. With HGH replacement therapy, the shrinkage that these organs undergo is checked, and in many cases, reversed, depending on which organ is involved and how early the intervention with HGH. Needless to say, once the HGH levels have reached those common to people of middle age, the sooner treatment is begun, the better.

To get a more complete idea of just how effective HGH is in this area, it would behoove us to examine its work on our inner organs in a bit more detail.

The Heart

The old song says "You Gotta Have Heart", and it's true. If your heart were to suddenly give out on you, you would be dead within minutes. That's how important the heart is.

Given the importance of the heart, you would think people would do what they could to keep it strong and healthy. Sadly, this is not the case. For decades, heart disease has been the leading cause of death in America.

Of late, many people have taken to looking after that crucial organ: cutting down on fats, going out jogging or walking, and so on. Even still, the years catch up. The heart is a muscle and it must beat up to 100,000 times a day, which works out to a few billion times throughout the average life span - without a rest. Although heart muscle is a different kind of muscle from our skeletal muscles, it is, like them, made up of cells - cells that eventually lose the ability to maintain and repair themselves with age. Even with proper diet and exercise. But this aging of the heart, as with much else in the body, can be slowed - and in many cases, reversed - by keeping HGH levels to where they were in our younger years.

At Sahlgrenska Hospital in Sweden, a study done by Bengt-Ake Bengtssön showed that patients with an HGH deficiency had twice the normal mortality rate as did those with normal HGH levels, when matched for age and sex. These were patients that also carried risk factors for cardiovascular disease such as higher cholesterol and triglyceride levels, as well as being overweight. The extra fat carried by these patients tended to be concentrated in and around the abdomen, the Tweedledumb fat. As we have seen, HGH is very effective in promoting fat loss of this sort. In so doing, HGH is also effective in promoting heart health.

HGH is also effective in promoting heart health in a more direct way. Just as it simulates the body to refurbish and rebuild skeletal muscles, so too it does for heart muscle. A study in Italy demonstrated this very well in a patient suffering from a weakened heart. After a short period of HGH therapy, this patient was observed - by means of echocardiography - to have made gains in the muscle mass of the left ventricle.

The left ventricle is the largest of the heart's chambers, and the one that pumps blood to the rest of the body, other than the lungs. When the left ventricle, and the rest of the heart, is made stronger, it is less likely to be overtaxed, less likely to provide inadequate blood supplies to other parts of the body. And less likely to fail.

In Dr. Chein's words, "Studies consistently show that growth hormone therapy increases left ventricular end-systolic dimension, stroke volume, and left ventricular mass." One of our colleagues recently rushed to the Intensive Care Unit (ICU) where his 90 year old father had suffered from his first heart attack.

His heart failure, not responding to maximal doses of Furosemide and other cardiac medications, responded to HGH and his father was discharged home.

Just as impressive is the effect that HGH may have in preventing cell death in the heart after heart attack or stroke.

In one study, heart attacks were produced in three groups of rats, after which each group was given one of three treatments: growth hormone, IGF-1, or placebo. Afterwards, when autopsies were performed on the rats, the two groups that had received either growth hormone or IGF-1 showed much less tissue death than did the group that had received the placebo. However studies on rats given supra physiological doses of GH, decrease longevity as anticipated.

HGH is beneficial to the heart-vascular system in yet another way, through its effect on cholesterol levels. Earlier we saw the potential of HGH for reducing the blood levels of undesired substances such as cholesterol. Cholesterol is a substance that is a major contributor to atherosclerosis, the buildup of plaque on the walls of arteries. Two of its components, HDL (high-density lipoprotein) and LDL (low-density lipoprotein), tend to work in opposite ways, one good, the other bad. The LDL is the bad one, and to help you remember, you might think of the "L" as standing for "lethal". HDL is the good one and as an additional mnemonic, you might think of the "H" as standing for "healthy".

It is the LDL that attaches itself to the walls of arteries, forming the plaque that gums up and partially blocks the arteries. This means that the blood has to be pumped through a narrower vessel, which means that blood flow will be impeded, and may give rise to hypertension.

It is the HDL that works against the buildup of LDL plaque on arterial walls. Bengtsson, in one of his studies, found that HGH tended to promote lower levels of LDL (the bad one) while increasing levels of HDL (the good one). The major consequence of this, one would expect, should be a reduced buildup of plaque on arterial walls. **Oxidative stress** has been shown to be a major factor in end organ damage with hypertension.

In a sense, then, HGH has shown itself to be a triple threat against heart disease: it strengthens the heart muscle itself; it appears (thus far) to reduce cell death in the heart that normally follows a heart attack (should we be unfortunate enough to have one); and it lowers the bad cholesterol that tends to collect on arterial walls and obstruct blood flow.

From the Heart

Coleridge wrote, "What comes from the heart, goes to the heart." No doubt he was referring to the flow of sentiment in poetry when he wrote those words. But their meaning may also hold a certain literal validity, as well, with respect to blood flow. For, the blood coming from the heart also goes to the heart - it feeds the coronary arteries, which supply the heart, itself, with blood. And these arteries are crucial. It is when these arteries becomes blocked that we have a so called heart attack.

This is why it is so important to keep the bad cholesterol at normal levels. And why it is important, therefore, to maintain HGH levels in a healthy, youthful range. Because statistically, when we do bring our HGH levels into this range, we tend to lower the levels of LDL or bad cholesterol in the blood. Lower LDL levels mean less plaque buildup, and down the road, less chance of a heart attack.

Because heart attack is so sudden, and so often final, the benefits of HGH are perhaps most obvious in this area of application. Certainly its use in countering heart disease is one of the better reasons for maintaining youthful levels of HGH in the blood. Because when we have good HGH levels, good things come from the heart.

The Lungs

The lungs work in conjunction with the heart in ridding the body of carbon dioxide and water, and most importantly, in bringing the body oxygenated blood. Every time we take a breath we are supplying the blood, and thence the rest of the body, with oxygen. And we do this thousands of times a day, without even thinking about it. Until something goes wrong.

One of the things that goes wrong is that we get older. (Although considering the alternative, that's not altogether bad.) As we get older, we have more trouble breathing. Sadly for some, a point is reached where they do think about every breath.

There is a test that is commonly used to tell how well we are able to breathe. It is called the forced expiratory volume test, or FEV1. It measures the volume of air, after filling our lungs fully, that we are able to force out in one second. Because the FEV1 test correlates so well with age, it is considered to be one of the more reliable indicators in predicting how long a person may expect to live, in the absence of chronic lung disease.

One study done by Cuneo and colleagues looked at how HGH treatment affected exercise capacity. For those who showed a deficiency in HGH levels, an oxygen uptake of only 80% of normal was all they could muster. After HGH therapy, their oxygen uptake had moved into the normal range. Also, their exercise capacity came into the normal range as well, especially for exercise that was carried out at below maximum output. This meant that they could now perform everyday tasks with normal ease.

In another study by Bengtsson and Rosen, patients who were deficient in pituitary function, and diminished lung capacity, were put on HGH for a year. At the end of this time the deterioration in lung capacity had been reversed, suggesting that HGH may confer "long term beneficial effects on pulmonary function."

Preliminary research into the effects of HGH on emphysema patients is so far very encouraging, and further positive data is expected in the future.

All of this evidence suggests that, since HGH has shown positive effects in treating those who, one way or another, were impaired in their vital capacity, it should promote the continued good health in lungs that are not yet impaired. All of which makes HGH replacement therapy for those entering middle age all the more attractive, for it will almost certainly be of help in their maintaining a healthy vital capacity farther into their golden years. Some of our Chronic Obstructive Lung Disease (COPD) patients have improved exercise tolerance with raised IGF-1 levels. Studies have demonstrated improved pulmonary function with HGH.

The Kidneys

The kidneys also work in conjunction with the heart, in this case, to cleanse the blood the heart pumps to the rest of the body. The kidneys filter out metabolic impurities and waste products from the blood, waste products such as urea.

Each kidney is made up of nephrons and tubules, which at one end have a concentration of intertwined capillaries (the glomerulus), and at the other, an opening into the interior cavity of the kidney itself. Each tubule consists of various sections along its length which carry out various filtration functions, straining out waste and returning much of the water back to the body. At its end stage, the "finished" urine is emptied into the kidney's central cavity, and from there to the bladder. Other than when we are signaled by a full bladder, we are never aware of this complex process. Until, as with the lungs, something goes wrong.

This something can be anything from injury, to disease, to cellular impairment brought on by the decay of age. Boxers who have suffered "kidney punches" are sometimes made aware of kidney injury by blood in the urine. Other problems with the kidneys may be determined by means of various tests. Where kidney failure is very pronounced, a patient may have to go on dialysis.

Just as the FEV1 test of the lungs was a reliable indicator of life expectancy, so too the kidneys may be tested to get a prediction about life expectancy from their perspective.

With the kidneys, as with the lungs, much of the data on HGH therapy comes from studies done on people who were already experiencing kidney problems.

One study on animals, conducted at the Harbor - UCLA Medical Center, showed that rats with an HGH deficiency achieved normalized glomerular function after undergoing HGH therapy. These rats also showed an increase in kidney weight, suggesting a restoration of structure that enabled the restoration of function.

Further, since HGH has the ability to counter toxins directly, this lessens the amount of nitrogenous waste in the blood, meaning there will be less of it that the kidneys have to filter out. Where kidney impairment is severe, or where other stresses are already affecting the body (as in burn or trauma patients, or the wasting of the body in the elderly), this assist to the kidneys is of immense value - as attested to by Dr. Chein, "In several studies involving kidney failure patients, human growth hormone's anticatabolic assistance was a lifesaver."

A study that further bears this out was conducted at the Tokyo Women's Medical College in Japan. Here, malnourished patients suffering from end-stage renal disease were treated with HGH. Those receiving HGH showed a greater improvement in their nutritional state than the control group, which did not receive HGH. With this improved nutrient uptake, an improved survival rate would also be expected.

Although much of the data concerning the effects of HGH on the kidney deals with kidneys that are already in a state of malfunction, it does strongly suggest that HGH replacement therapy for those going into middle age should retard some of the prospective effects of aging in the kidney. Amino acid secretogogues may be difficult for a renal or kidney failure patient to handle, and these patients are treated as special cases.

The Liver

The liver is the largest organ of the body, not counting the skin. It is something like a complex production plant or factory in the body. One of its main functions is the conversion of sugar into lipids and carbohydrates, which it then stores for use between meals. It also breaks down aging red blood cells that need to be removed from service. The liver not only takes LDL out of the blood, but makes it. Some of the material the liver removes from the blood is used in its production of bile, which is passed on to the gall bladder, and from there to the intestines, where it assists in the digestion of fats.

Since HGH stimulates LDL receptor sites in the liver, it improves liver function in removing LDL from the blood. Also, since HGH is instrumental in bringing about repair work in cells both directly and as IGF-1, it is effective in stimulating liver cells to repair themselves. This is particularly important because if the liver is not working up to par, a greater burden falls on the kidneys, eventually overtaxing them in their job.

Numerous studies have shown this "healing" effect of HGH on the liver. However, whenever liver damage is extreme, whether from injury, disease, or the over-consumption of alcohol, the restorative effects of HGH are considerably diminished. As Dr. Chein has stated, "...the anabolic properties of growth hormone positively affects protein metabolism, suggesting that GH therapy could be used to treat those with chronic liver disease."

For the liver, as for other parts of the body, the watchword is prevention. If we begin maintaining optimal HGH levels before we come to poor health, there is the increased likelihood that we will not come to poor health.

The Brain

Malcolm Cowley once stated: "They tell you that you'll lose your mind when you grow older. What they don't tell you is that you won't miss it very much."

In looking at patients with Alzheimer's Disease one might be strongly inclined to disagree with Cowley's observation.

For centuries philosophers have debated the mind-body aspect of our existence. At present science marshals an immense body of evidence to show that we - our minds, our personalities, our identities - all tend to derive from the existence, structure, and biochemistry of the brain. If we lose an arm or a leg, of course we become changed. But the root core of our identity generally remains intact. But if it is the brain that is seriously damaged, very often this root core of our identity does becomes altered.

As people age, we frequently see changes in them. Often, the thought processes appear to slow down at some point. Farther along still, and memory, too, is affected, becoming fuzzy, patchy. In some extreme cases a point is reached where there is little or nothing left of an individual's identity.

We have seen how HGH brings about marvelous effects on other parts of the body - promoting repair, stopping or reversing shrinkage in organs, and so on. Because it works at the cellular level, HGH is also able to confer beneficial effects on the brain and nerve tissue. However, where HGH can promote healing and regrowth in other tissues and cells, it is not able to bring about regrowth in nerve cells. Nothing, so far, has been able to, although there is promising research in this area. But because HGH has been shown to increase nerve growth factors, it appears at least possible that by raising HGH levels to an optimal point, we can bring about a rebuilding of brain cells.

For example, although researchers have not been able, by the use of HGH therapy, to bring about the growth of new nerve cells, they have been able to induce renewed dendritic connections, which are the spidery-like arms that connect the neurons for communication. Also, since the glial cells, which are brain cells that nourish the neurons, are capable of being renewed, HGH may well have a positive impact on that front. This certainly suggests an avenue of fruitful research for the future.

A recent study conducted by Barbara Johnston, Peter Gluckman, and colleagues at the University of Auckland, New Zealand, demonstrated a striking result for IGF-1, the form in which HGH does much of its work. Injecting IGF-1 into brain injured fetal lambs, they were able to save damaged neurons. As well, they were able to stave off apoptosis - the programmed death of cells - in these brain injured lambs. Apoptosis is generally thought to be an accompanying result from such brain injury, a result that may continue to take its toll for up to three days following the injury. The IGF-1 injections prevented these anticipated cell deaths.

HGH has also been shown to bring about increased concentrations of neurotransmitters in the brain. Since these neurotransmitters are the actual carriers of information from brain cell to brain cell, one would expect HGH to speed up and enhance brain function. And many who have undergone HGH replacement therapy have attested to just that: they've got back the sharp memory of younger days, recaptured the quick thinking. To quote Dr. Chein once again: "Loss of memory has long been linked to aging, and now, researchers have found a direct link between memory skills and the amount of growth hormone in the body."

One of Dr. Chein's own studies, done with Dr. Terry at Palm Springs, supports this strongly. In that study, 62% of patients reported an improvement in memory.

To date, the results of HGH on brain structure and function have all been positive. And although HGH has not led researchers to the holy grail of neural research - the regeneration of neurons - it has shown many beneficial effects. Most importantly, HGH has shown that it may be effective in helping us to maintain our identity, to remain who we have always been as we go through the aging process.

The Bones

"If it ain't broke, don't fix it."

That may sound like good advice. Except, of course, if what ain't broke actually is broke, but it ain't visible.

For example, where people are undernourished

throughout a good part of their lives, they will tend to have a shorter life span than would have occurred with optimal nutrition. So although the problem here wasn't immediately apparent, it was one that did need to be fixed.

Many post-menopausal women are at risk for osteoporosis. Here again, there is no obvious problem, nothing that is in apparent need of being fixed. Nothing, that is, until the bone density diminishes to the point at which a slight bump or slip is enough to cause a broken hip or pelvis. But by then it may be too late, because fixing the problem at that stage will not be so easy.

We tend to take our bones for granted. They are hidden away inside the flesh, out of sight. Yet they are so necessary, providing a framework for the body and a protective cage of sorts for the vital organs within. But out of sight though they may be, age is ever working on our bones.

When we are young our bones are growing and strengthening, doing so at the bidding of osteoblasts, which are bone growth stimulators. This brings about the growth of children into adults. Past the age of thirty, our bones are subject to a preponderance of osteoclasts, which promote bone absorption. During much of adulthood, the two are in approximate balance. However, once we get into middle age and the balance has shifted strongly in favor of the osteoclasts, the bones undergo a sort of "leaching". They lose more minerals still. For some, as old age is approached , the bones have become extremely weak and brittle, a condition indicative of the disease called osteoporosis. In this condition bones can snap like a dry twig.

We have seen how HGH was first used to promote

growth in children with pituitary deficiencies. Other studies have since shown that HGH levels tend to correlate very closely with bone density. One such study done in Germany indicated that adults deficient in HGH showed only a 51% bone mass density in the lumbar vertebrae when measured against those with normal HGH levels. For the forearm, the figure was 73%.

We have seen from Dr. Rudman's study of HGH replacement therapy in elderly males, that there was an average 1.6% increase in the bone mass density of the lumbar vertebrae. Studies since have corroborated these findings.

Healthy, strong bones are the key to our going into our golden years with grace. Healthy bones often mean the difference between sitting idly by, whiling away the endless hours, creaking almost audibly when we do hobble about, or being able to participate in a variety of activities, like swimming, golf, or travel. HGH provides the choice, but the choice is yours to make. Recently Dr. Bart Swierstra from Rotterdam showed that increased IGF-1 levels improved hip fracture recovery among 111 females over the age of 60 years. Hormone replacement with estrogens, progesterone and testosterone - in conjunction with proper nutrition - have shown benefits in the treatment of osteoporosis. Medications simulating human calcitonin and recently some cholesterol lowering medications are being used to improve osteoporosis (thinning bones).

The Beef

We have already touched upon the fine job HGH does in beefing up the muscles. Still, the topic deserves a few more words.

As with fat loss, muscle gain is a result that can readily be observed, without complex scientific measurement and testing; and to carry out such testing might strike some as on a par with a person sitting out on the patio, and listening to the radio to find out what the weather is doing. In any case, researchers, being the curious lot they are, have scrutinized the effects of HGH in the field of muscle gain. And persiflage and joshing aside, the research does bear out what the eye has seen.

An early study by D.B. Cheek and D. E. Hill back in the 60's gave an early indication of muscle mass gain exhibited by HGH therapy. Other studies since, building on Bengtssön's study at Sahlgrenska and Dr. Rudman's initial study in the U.S., all indicate strongly that HGH replacement therapy consistently brings about gains in muscle mass.

The study done by Cheek and Hill suggests that HGH brings about increases in muscle mass by stimulating an increase in the number of muscle cells, as opposed to merely increasing the size of the cells. Bengtssön's study, which showed a 6% increase in body cell mass after one year of HGH treatment, does tend to support this conclusion.

There is further evidence to attest to muscle mass gains that perhaps in some cases the eye cannot see - biochemical evidence. We have in our bodies a white crystalline compound, creatinine, which is produced mainly in the muscles as a result of metabolic activity. Measurements of how much creatinine is passed out of the body in the urine during a 24 hour period, correlate well with the quantity of muscle mass in the body, provided the kidneys are healthy. In a study done by

F. Salomon et al, the amount of creatinine collected in a 24 hour period was higher after HGH therapy, indicating biochemically that an increase in muscle mass was taking place.

Again, we might liken this testing to the guy on the patio with the radio...but it is always nice to have scientific corroboration.

Happily, the agreement between science and the eye indicates that HGH does bring about bigger, stronger muscles. Moreover, as with fat loss, it produces this result without a change in diet or exercise. One might imagine, however, that once people see the fat dropping away and the muscles growing and firming up, that it just might be the motivation needed to improve their dietary and exercise regime. Because now, at last, they can see that progress is possible.

Heal!

It would make sense that if HGH promotes cell regrowth and repair, and if HGH rejuvenates organs that have been atrophying and shrinking, and if HGH brings about increases in muscle mass, then it should also help to speed and enhance the healing of wounds. And that is exactly the case.

Early evidence of this goes back to the 1960's, where HGH was first administered to patients recovering from wounds resulting from surgery or injury. Since then, numerous studies and publications have attested to the beneficial effects of HGH on wound healing. Further, HGH has been particularly useful where healing is difficult and crucial: severe burns, trauma injuries, skin grafts, and the like. In experiments done in Japan recently, burn victims have shown the improvement expected with increased IGF-1 levels.

Since HGH works at the cellular level, it assists the healing process on internal injuries and external injuries alike. Where an injured part or limb must be kept immobilized, often there is an accompanying wasting or atrophying in the tissues. Because HGH strengthens and builds muscle even in the absence of exercise, it has been particularly effective in minimizing the wasting and weakening of muscle tissue when it has been immobilized. In so doing, HGH has demonstrated a capacity to accelerate recovery, and to reduce the amount of physiotherapy required after the initial healing.

Studies on animals have produced similar good results. One study conducted in Denmark involved rats with experimental colitis. The rats that received HGH treatments were observed to exhibit less damage - both at the macroscopic and microscopic levels - than did the control group. Further, these rats were able to come back to their original body weight after only 7 days of treatment. The control group, on the other hand, still weighed in at 11% below their original weight at the end of this period.

In other studies on animals, observations indicate that HGH has been able to promote healing on internal surgery as well. One study, in which lengthy segments of the digestive tract were surgically removed, showed that actual regeneration of the digestive tract had taken place after HGH treatments. Also in this study, HGH was shown to increase the speed of recovery. All of which suggests that for humans undergoing serious gastrointestinal surgery in the future, HGH may well be chosen to assist them in their recovery. Burn victims have shown the improvement expected with increased IGF-1 levels on experiments done in Japan recently.

Sex

We humans are one of the sexiest animals on earth. Women do not have an annual estrus as do many mammals, but ovulate every month. Men, in their prime at least, are pretty much ready anytime. Further, where most animals copulate for the purpose of reproduction, humans copulate largely for pleasure.

One theory to account for this phenomenon is that it came about because of the helplessness of the newborn human, and the lengthy period of training the infant needed until it could fend for itself. This meant that its chances of survival were greater if the male stayed with the female in something of a pair bond. That way, the male would share in the feeding and the protection of the young through its period of training and development.

To effect this pair bond, however loose it may have been at times, some anthropologists theorize that we evolved a biology that entailed the possibility of ongoing and frequent sexual activity as an enticement, which may even have led to what we now regard as romantic love. This kept the couple together and increased the survival chances of the offspring.

Whatever its origins, the current propensity of humans for frequent sexual activity is undeniable. And most often, when this propensity begins to fade with age, there is a certain sadness in us. Because, up to this point, frequent sexual activity has, over the years, been a source of pleasure for most of us, and for some, a source of love renewal and soul bonding. And as we get on in years, as we feel the drive slipping away, the intensity dying off, it is like the tolling of a bell for what has been a beautiful aspect of our lives.

Harder, Faster

That sex is a very important aspect of our lives is attested to by the roaring sales of Viagra since its release, bought up by men who wanted to rekindle the embers in the sexual furnace, to refuel the fire. The drug has been so much in demand that there is talk that an equivalence of it will eventually become available to women.

An alternative solution to the problem, one which confers a great many other benefits in addition to refueling the sexual fires, is HGH replacement therapy. Sexual renewal, along with fat loss and muscle gain, is one of the most consistent findings reported for HGH. And at a fraction of the cost, HGH enhancement through secretogogues might be looked upon as the poor man's Viagra.

Sexual Dysfunction in Men

For men in general, the cause of impotence is nowadays thought to have an underlying physical basis in about 75% of cases. For men over 50, that figure jumps to 90%. Also for men over 50, almost one half of erectile dysfunction is due to arteriosclerosis of the penile arteries. The buildup of plaque in the penile arteries involves the similar kinds of plaque that clog the walls of other arteries, including the coronary arteries.

J. E. Morley has indicated, in an article in Postgraduate Medicine, that such erectile dysfunction may serve as an indicator for future heart attack or stroke.

We have seen that HGH has been instrumental in reducing cholesterol levels in the blood, particularly LDL, the component that contributes most to the buildup of plaque on artery walls. Although research has yet to confirm it definitively, with the reduction of LDL in the blood, one would tend to conclude that it would reduce the plaque buildup in the penile arteries. There is a theory relating to the finite number of sexual encounters in one lifetime allowed by oxidative stress.

Further, some of the main risk factors for heart disease, such as smoking, high cholesterol (especially LDL) levels, high triglyceride levels, also comprise some of the same risk factors for impotence. If we revisit the study done at Palm Springs, we will recall that a figure of 75% was reported for improvement in sexual potency and frequency by over 200 patients in that study. Since HGH has shown itself, in this study and others, to confer remarkable improvements in patients' sex lives, and since HGH has also shown itself to be efficacious in ameliorating conditions often attendant with poor sex lives, such as high cholesterol and high triglycerides, could it be that HGH is working on the physiological root cause of both? Or working on something that is at least a partial root cause of both?

Whatever the ultimate physiological explanation, the main point is that HGH has been shown to effect a striking improvement in both sexual satisfaction and performance. Although few studies have focused specifically on the effects of HGH in this area, a number of researchers have commented on reports made by patients in this regard. Bengt-Ake Bengtssön had a number of patients from one study report an improvement in sex drive and performance. Also, many patients asked to be allowed to continue with HGH therapy once the study was completed.

Dr. Terry, as we will recall, first contacted Dr. Chein about losing fat around his (Dr. Terry's) middle, and was put on HGH. Besides the positive results already recorded in this regard, Dr. Terry also experienced the sexual boost that so many others have attested to. The effects were so pronounced that even his wife was amazed. As Dr. Terry jokingly put it,"It scared my wife. She said, 'What's that doctor doing to you?'"

This experience is fairly typical of patients who have received HGH treatment for one reason, and to their pleasant surprise, found that their sex life had been greatly improved as well.

Sexual Dysfunction in Women

As for problems that women encounter in the area of sex, at first glance it may appear that they are not as drastic as those that afflict men. After all, nothing shuts down sexual intercourse faster than a flaccid penis. Nevertheless, the problems faced by some women in this area are just as serious.

One of these problems can take the form of vaginal dryness. A situation where vaginal secretions are not occurring at normal levels, while perhaps not preclusive of intercourse altogether, may certainly cause pain and discomfort. Which may cause a woman to avoid sex. Or which may, at the very least, elicit from a woman the same attitude toward sex as reflected in a response made (purportedly) by a British lady from the prissy Victorian era, when asked how she managed to endure the act: "I just lay back and think of England."

Most would agree that sex should involve something more than thoughts of England. Further, painful intercourse will inevitably entail other problems. Almost certainly it will lead to an avoidance of sex. That is because, if the situation is not corrected, all too often the eventual course is no intercourse. This can leave a woman feeling inadequate or incomplete, just as erectile dysfunction does for a man, and it can put heavy strains on a marriage or relationship.

As is the case for men, diminished desire is one of the more common problems experienced by women as they age. Although not as prohibitive to a continued sex life as lack of lubrication, lack of desire does reduce something that had been truly exciting to something that is humdrum, relegating the act of "lovemaking" to that of "duty".

Accompanying the diminished desire that often comes to women as they approach middle age, is a corresponding diminished level of estrogen and testosterone. And HGH. While estrogen replacement therapy has shown that it can help correct vaginal dryness, and testosterone, progesterone and DHEA have been able to bring back some of the lost desire, the strongest effects in this area have been brought about by HGH.

Replacement therapy with HGH has shown consistently good, and sometimes even spectacular, results. As was the case for men, many women undergoing HGH treatment have experienced a total rejuvenation in their sex lives. Some have reported a complete recapturing of their youthful, lusty libido; others, a renewed vigor and energy, and more intense orgasms; others still, reporting that they now achieve multiple orgasms.

An added benefit conferred by HGH is that it has shown, in a number of cases, a capacity to ease or eliminate problems associated with menstrual cycles and menopause, alleviating conditions such as PMS and hot flashes. For the latter, the Palm Springs study showed a 58% improvement, while menstrual cycle regulation showed a 39% improvement.

Size Does Matter

And then there's the one about what Adam said when he first laid eyes on Eve: "Stand back! I don't know how big this thing gets."

The reason the line is funny is that we know how big the thing gets. Within limits. But within these limits there is room for considerable variance. And when we hear someone say "Size doesn't matter." it is usually said by a woman. So long as a penis is not too far off average, for most women, size does not matter. But to most men, size does matter. And it matters a lot. For a man, that part of him is his bowsprit, his figurehead. He wants to be proud of it.

Just as many organs, such as the heart or liver, tend to shrink with age, so too for the penis. (And the clitoris, too, for that matter.) As we get into our forties and fifties, the shrinkage for some can be somewhat pronounced. But here again HGH can help. Just as HGH has shown that it can stop, and in many cases reverse, the shrinkage in various inner organs, so too it can halt and reverse shrinkage in the penis.

A study done by the Mayo Clinic on HGH deficient men showed that HGH alone was able to restore the penis to its normal size.

This corroborates findings by Dr. Chein, who wrote, "When you restore the hormones to that of a 20 year old, the man's penis and the woman's clitoris will return to their original size. This has not been reported in the journals yet, but these are the results from my patients after six month, one year, two years, and longer."

For a man in his forties or fifties, it is bad enough to be hit with a diminishing libido. Finding that the penis has begun to shrink as well, has to be a case of insult being added to injury, a double whammy. Happily, HGH has a one-two punch in its repertoire to take on the diminishing libido and the shrinking penis.

Just as HGH turns back the clock for the rest of the body, so too it does for the penis. It allows a man to recapture his former drive and his former size. It allows him to stand proud and stand tall, and to say: "Stand back!"

The Rebuilt Engine

As we approach middle age, many of us have put on those extra pounds around the middle, and have allowed muscles to soften and go slack. Also, in arranging our livelihoods and furthering our careers, we have frequently put ourselves through years of stress. All of which takes a toll on our sex lives.

Yogi Berra once said "Ninety percent of baseball is half mental." The same could be said for sex. Sort of.

That is to say, a good deal of our libido derives from just how our minds are predisposed to sex at any given time. If we feel flabby and unattractive, if we are out of shape and out of energy, sex will likely be out of the question. And out of the picture.

Because HGH can and does work on several fronts at once, it can and does put sex back into the picture. Once HGH has begun to trim us down and fill out the muscles, we begin to feel better about our bodies, and our attractiveness. It has been said that a woman's greatest asset is a man's imagination. Of course, the vice-versa is true as well. And once we feel we have attained sufficient attractiveness to inflame our partner's imagination, our frozen assets can readily be converted to liquid assets, and we are now into a bull market, so to speak.

As we have mentioned previously, HGH begins its rejuvenating work in the cells, in the tissues, and in the organs, working throughout the body. In this comprehensive rejuvenation almost everything in the body is affected by repair and restoration. HGH does not just induce a short term Viagra fix. It makes our cells and tissues younger, it halts the shrinking in many of our internal organs - it even brings shrinking genitals back to normal. And it is all done by bringing back a more youthful physiology throughout. Which is why we lose the fat and gain the muscle. Which is why we experience higher energy levels. Which is why we experience a more buoyant frame of mind. (Remember the increased levels of beta-endorphins?)

So it's not surprising that, with this comprehensive rejuvenation taking place, that the sex organs, too, are rejuvenated. As well as the desire. Particularly the desire.

Restoring HGH to normal levels is the equivalent of taking a used racing car engine and giving it a complete rebuild: ring job, valve job, carburetor overhaul, new spark plugs - the works. Of course, once the engine has had its worn parts replaced or retooled, and all painstakingly put back in place, the engine is bound to work like new, like it just came off the assembly line - ready for the Indianapolis 500.

Little wonder, then, at the effect HGH has had on people who have undergone treatment - their improved physical appearance, their renewed enthusiasm, their enriched and turbo-charged sex lives. It's as though they've had their engines overhauled and rebuilt. It's as though they, too, feel like new, like they just came off the assembly line. And like the rebuilt racing car, they too are once again ready for the Indianapolis 500.

So...Ladies and gentlemen: Start Your Engines!

The Endocrine System

The endocrine system consists of various ductless glands that produce hormones. They are called ductless glands because they produce substances - in this case, hormones - that are secreted directly into the blood. These hormones, which act as chemical messengers, are generally quite specific as to the effects they bring about. The thyroid, for example, through its hormones thyroxine (T4) and triiodothyronine (T3), regulates the general metabolic level at which the body's cells operate. The adrenal glands produce adrenalin and steroids which girds the body for action during fight or flight situations.

HGH, on the other hand, operates in a much broader fashion, and on several fronts at once. One very important function of HGH is that it increases the efficiency of receptor sites on a great many cells in the body. These receptor sites are where hormones attach to a cell to stimulate it to effect a particular activity. By making these receptor sites more "receptive", HGH improves the efficacy of other hormones in achieving their intended results.

We might compare the body's hormones to tradesmen or contractors on a construction site. These hormones, like plumbers or carpenters, perform fairly specific tasks. In contrast, HGH might be likened to a master builder or general contractor. Just as a general contractor facilitates the work of plumbers or carpenters at various sites on the construction project, so too HGH facilitates the work of the other hormones at the sites of their operation.

HGH also affects the performance of the various endocrine glands themselves, and is able, in Dr. Chein's words "...to bring production of other hormones up to optimal levels. This feature works both ways, in fact, demonstrating that all hormones work synergistically with each other. If DHEA, melatonin, and estrogen are all at their optimal levels, they can stimulate the pituitary gland to produce and secrete a greater amount of HGH, restoring it to a more optimal level."

This interrelationship is most pronounced between HGH and thyroid hormone. Studies have shown that where levels of thyroid hormone are low, usually HGH levels are low as well. When the levels of HGH are raised with replacement therapy, there is a corresponding improvement in thyroid function.

Since HGH has shown such a widespread effect, not only on the cells and organs of the body, but on the endocrine system in general, maintaining optimal levels of HGH as we get on in years, will almost certainly provide an assist to the other hormones as well. Further, maintaining our youthful levels of HGH is one of the simplest ways of promoting our hormonal health. Because, if it is true that a rising tide raises all ships, HGH is most certainly that rising tide.

The Immune System

In his book "Stopping The Clock", Dr. Ronald Klatz has listed his rules for Immortality. Rule #1 is: Don't Die. And in case that doesn't cover the matter fully, Rule #2 is: Don't Get Sick.

Obviously, if we observe Rule #2 we will promote the observance of Rule #1. And an important way of promoting the observance of both rules is to maintain a vigorous immune system.

With the advent of AIDS, almost everyone has by now heard of the immune system. The immune system consists of numerous entities in our bodies, chiefly components in the blood and the lymphatics, that protect us against disease.

If we look at some of the effects of AIDS on people - the wasting, the diminishing ability to fight off disease, we see that in some respects Aids parallels aging, except that with aging, the effects manifest themselves over a longer period of time. As with Aids, aging brings on a general deterioration of the body. Accompanying this is a deterioration in the immune system, which in our later years, leaves us vulnerable to infections like pneumonia and flu. In our younger years, girded with a strong immune system, we usually fight these infections off within a week or two. But in our later years, with a weakened immune system, it is often the infections that win.

Natural Born Killers

There are microscopic things that try to kill us. Usually these are bacteria or viruses, but they may even be cells of our own bodies, such as out-of-control cancer cells. And then there are things in us that try to kill them. These are our natural born killers.

These natural born killers, white blood cells or leukocytes, originate in the marrow of long bones (along with our red blood cells), and as well, in the lymph nodes and the thymus gland. Members of this protective army include, neutrophils, NK (natural killer) cells, and T-cells. Each of these serves to protect us against different threats. The neutrophils, for instance, engulf foreign invaders of almost any kind. The NK cells, battle against would-be cancer cells. The T-cells specialize in taking on viruses, and it is the T-cells that are at the forefront of this army of natural born killers.

Stem Cells, Progenitor Cells

The T-cells, along with all the other red and white blood cells, develop from cells in the marrow called stem cells. The stem cells, in turn, evolve into progenitor cells. It is the progenitor cells that differentiate into the various red and white blood cells.

A researcher at the University of Illinois at Urbana-Champaign, Dr. Keith Kelley, has found, in some of his most recent work, that the progenitor cells in both older humans and older rodents, were in serious decline. When he gave growth hormone to the old rats, the progenitor cells showed a marked resurgence and regained their numbers.

Since stem cells have the capacity to outlast the human life span, Dr. Kelley believes that the problem of diminished progenitor cells does not originate with the stem cells, but elsewhere in the production line. There is some mechanism in the production line that becomes blocked or defunct with age. But whatever that blocked mechanism is, growth hormone is able to help set it right. In Dr. Kelley's words "Somehow the hormones act to overcome a block...We don't know exactly what happens. Magic occurs."

No doubt the details of this striking discovery are currently being sought out through further research. Meanwhile, this "magic" leaves us with an irresistible chain of logic: Humans and rodents suffer diminished immune capacity as they age. And as they age humans and rodents suffer diminished numbers of progenitor cells (which are the cells that give rise to our army of disease fighters). Growth hormone brings back the number of progenitor cells in aging rodents. Therefore, since growth hormone does strengthen the human immune system, it seems likely that one way in which it does this is by bringing back the numbers of progenitor cells in aging humans.

The Thymus

Perhaps the most striking discovery made by Dr. Kelley has to do with the thymus gland.

The thymus gland is something of an anomaly.

Located behind the upper part of the breastbone, the thymus is at its largest size in childhood. As physicians, we are amazed by the huge size of the thymus in the newborn chest x-ray. Almost from the time of birth the thymus begins to shrink, and by age sixty it has shriveled down to almost nothing. From the thymus gland are produced many thymus protein hormones such as the 500 amino acid Thymus Protein-A, discovered by Dr. Terry Berdsley in 1983. Many of these thymic proteins have shown promise in the treatment of Hepatitis A, Hepatitis C, AIDS, herpes, fungal infections and cancer. We are convinced that many of our cancer patients have improved with thymus stimulation as an adjunct to their conventional cancer treatment.

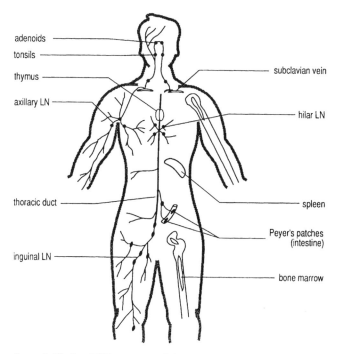

Lymph Nodes (LN) as part of the body's lymphatic system of drainage for immune function against cancer, toxins and infection showing relationship to Thymus.

The thymus has long been regarded as a principal player in the immune system. One of its most important functions is that it assists in the maturation of T-cells. These T-lymphocytes mature in the Thymus gland to become either helper cells (CD4 cells) or T-suppressor / killer cells (CD8 cells). The helper cells recognize the invaders and the killer cells destroy the invaders. Given that most of the shrinkage, or involution, of the thymus occurs from adulthood onward, and that the levels of HGH tend to decline during this same period, Dr. Kelley wondered if there was a connection between the two. Could HGH be a factor affecting the involution of the thymus?

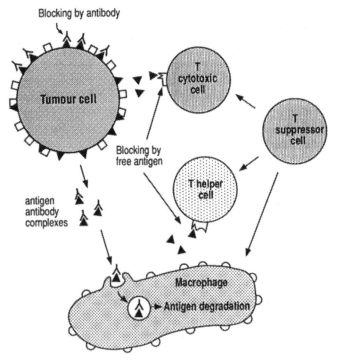

Defects preventing proper immune response to tumour showing different T-Cells, some programmed from the Thymus.

To answer this question he set up an experiment with old rats whose thymus glands had all but disappeared. He injected these rats with GH3 cells, which are cells that secrete large quantities of growth hormone. The experiment confirmed his intuition - with a stunning result. The thymus glands in the old rats were restored to the size they had been when the rats were young..

Prior to this experiment it had been almost universally held that the involution of the thymus was irreversible, that organisms were genetically programmed to lose the thymus, that it was inevitable. In Dr. Kelley's words: "Everyone considered that the thymus went away and you couldn't get it back. But clearly that was incorrect. It was not due to a genetic defect. It was not programmed to go away in the sense that you could not get it back. You could get it back by using a treatment. And that treatment is growth hormone."

As a corollary to this finding, Dr. Kelley also discovered that the T-cells in the treated rats were restored to where they were able to make more interleukin 2. "The synthesis of interleukin 2 by T-cells in old rats goes down. If you give them growth hormone, it comes back up."

You can almost hear a "Eureka!" in his words.

Other Fronts

Research concerning the effects of growth hormone on the immune system has been carried out on several fronts. One area of particular interest involves the work of Dr. Vincent Giampapa. Treating patients with HGH he has found improvements in T-cell function, in antibody synthesis, and in the cell division of lymphocytes. Most significantly, there was an improvement in two cancer fighters - tumor necrosis factor alpha, and NK (natural killer) cells. Dr. Giampapa also found HGH brought about a growth in the thymus as well as improved DNA synthesis of cells in the thymus.

An explanation of the latter finding is likely connected to another result in Dr. Giampapa's work, a study involving cell division. As part of a cell's existence, it goes through a quiescent stage, where it carries on its routine functions. Then, in another stage, the cell undergoes the process of cell division, during which some rejuvenation and repair of the cell takes place. With age, the quiescent phase grows longer, meaning that the periods between cell division and repair grow farther apart. What Dr. Giampapa found was that with HGH treatment, the periods of quiescence were reduced. "What growth hormone does is jump start the older cell," explains Dr. Giampapa. "Growth hormone pushes the cell so it goes into the repair and reproduction stage more quickly."

On yet another front comes another striking piece of information - this from research done by David Khansari and Thomas Gustad at North Dakota State University in Fargo. They treated older mice with growth hormone and obtained a startling result: growth hormone extended the life span of these mice by a full one third. The older mice treated with growth hormone also showed an improved production of immune factors such as tumor necrosis factor, interleukin 1, and immunoglobulin G. As well, these results tend to corroborate the thesis that the T-cells in aging animals are not innately defective, that they are capable of being rejuvenated by growth hormone.

Dr. Richard Aspinall at Imperial College School of

Medicine, London U.K., demonstrated that women have higher levels of new T-cells than men of the same age, which could explain women's better resistance to infection, and hence greater longevity.

Refortifying the Fort, Re-arming the Army

Our bodies are in perpetual combat against disease and death. When we are young our bodies are in good condition, like a newly built fort. As we age this fort falls into disrepair. However, HGH has shown that it can refortify the aging fort, to refurbish and rebuild much of it. Just as it restores and rebuilds cells and organs, it has also been shown that it can rebuild and restore elements of the bone marrow, and the thymus gland. With this rebuilt fort we are then better able to ward off and repel attacks from intruders such as bacteria and viruses - and even from saboteurs such as arthritis, and fifth columnists such as cancer cells.

In addition to the fort falling into disrepair as we age, the army within it ages as well. Our army of natural born killers - those battlers in our blood - become less deadly. This army also becomes less formidable in number. The attrition of the years takes its toll. The army has, to a considerable extent, become disarmed.

But here, too, HGH serves as an ally. It can re-arm the army. And while it has not shown that it can re-arm all aspects of our immune system, it has shown that it can re-arm a good deal of it. Besides the improvements growth hormone is able to bring to the bone marrow and the thymus, it has been shown to restore or improve the function of virus fighters such as T-cells, as well as cancer fighters such as NK cells, and to improve the production of other immune factors such as tumor necrosis factor and interleukin 1 and 2.

Most importantly, growth hormone has shown that it can restore the resupplying of progenitor cells that tend to decline with age. That is especially significant because the progenitor cells might be compared to the raw recruits at boot camp, and keeping their numbers high is crucial to keeping the rest of the army up to full strength.

Leaving off from the military metaphor at this point, we'll give Dr. Chein the last word on the topic. "The connection between HGH and the immune system goes beyond NK cells and the ability to combat cancerous tumors. Research has found a clear relationship between HGH levels and the body's ability to fend off any disease. HGH deficiency has been shown to cause, or at least contribute to immunodeficiency. So, HGH replacement is an effective therapy for improving the body's overall natural ability to defend itself against disease. Even if a person has enough of the NK cells and other immune system ammunition, there is experimental evidence to support that HGH therapy will enhance the activity of these, making them work even more quickly and efficiently to fight off infection and disease."

Additional Benefits

Besides the many benefits of HGH therapy that we have already looked at, there are others. Some of these include improved sleep, lower stress levels, and an increase in energy levels.

It may appear somewhat dismissive to have these benefits lumped together as "additional benefits" but that is certainly not the intent. Anyone who has had one or two sleepless nights, and then tried to function the next day, knows just how important a good night's sleep is. Just as important is having our stress levels and our energy levels in a comfortable range. When they are not, we may, at the least, experience very unpleasant days, and at the worst, considerable impairment.

Also, these aspects of our health often tie in together, so that when one suffers, they all suffer. For instance, when we are getting poor sleeps, usually our energy levels are low as well. Oftentimes, too, when our energy levels are low we feel the daily stresses more acutely. With higher stress levels we come full circle to poorer sleep. Each affects the other.

Unfortunately, aging tends to impact negatively on all of these areas, particularly our sleep. As we get on in years, we find we are less able to sleep through the night. And when we awaken, have greater difficulty falling back to sleep. Also, as we get older we tend to be less adaptable, and we frequently feel more intensely the stresses that in our youth we would have shrugged off without a thought. And we have all seen the drop in energy levels that generally tend to accompany middle age and beyond.

Happily, HGH has shown very strong positive effects in all of these areas.

A Good Night's Sleep

"Sleep that knits up the ravelled sleave of care...
Chief nourisher in life's feast."

Shakespeare knew how important a good night's sleep was. So do we, but usually it takes a night or two of poor sleep before we come to realize it fully.

When we are young, we can often race around all day, and when night comes, sleep like the dead, waking in the morning refreshed and alive - ready for another day filled with activity. As we age this changes.

Not only do we suffer more broken sleep as we get older, the quality of our sleep declines. We tend to sleep less deeply. Also, we tend to achieve less time in REM sleep, the sleep during which we dream.

REM sleep is acutely important to our mental health. One experiment in psychology showed that where experimental subjects were deprived of REM sleep (but were allowed to get enough sleep otherwise), they began to exhibit symptoms of mental illness, and for some, these symptoms extended even to the point where they began to hallucinate. When they were allowed to catch up on their REM sleep, these symptoms disappeared.

In addition to REM sleep there are four stages of sleep.

<u>Stage 1</u> is the drowsy time, where the body is in preparation for sleep, and where we still have some awareness of our surroundings. In this stage the brain waves are seen as theta waves, and from this early sleep we may be easily wakened.

<u>Stage 2</u> is the light sleep that is a low voltage sleep with brief bursts of activity known as sleep spindles and K-complexes.

<u>Stage 3</u> is a 15 minute period of true sleep before the deep sleep, and at this stage 50% of the EEG shows large voltage delta waves.

<u>Stage 4</u> is the deepest sleep. During this time most repair work is done by the body under the influence of maximal HGH secretion in men.

Mortality and Sleep: The Connection

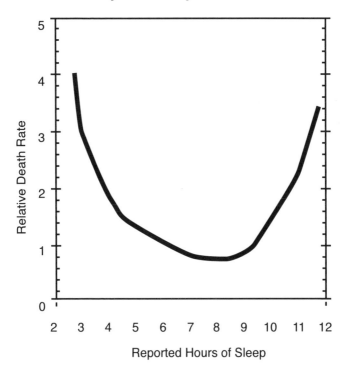

If we sleep the optimum 8 hours per night, then we have spent 200,000 hours in the sleep state by the age of 70 years. One colleague has remarked that if we could stay awake for just one extra hour each day, then we could have an extra 25,000 hours (about 3 years) of awake time. This could mean more reading time or more T.V. but could it also mean diminished secretions of HGH ??

As we saw earlier, when sleep is fitful and broken, we tend to secrete less HGH into the bloodstream at night, bringing on the unwanted cycle - poor sleep causing lower HGH levels, and lower HGH levels causing still poorer sleep. Dr. Eve Van Cauter, a sleep researcher at the University of Chicago, believes that if the capacity for deep sleep can be restored in people as they age, then the aging process may be slowed. Further, she feels that impaired HGH secretion caused by insomnia in older men is responsible for premature aging.

There are other problems, as well, associated with sleep deprivation, and since inadequate sleep is a widespread malady in the modern world, this compounds the problem. Approximately 100,000 traffic accidents and at least 1,500 deaths are attributed to sleep deprivation. Accidents at home and in the workplace are frequently caused by lack of proper sleep.

Common problems are insomnia (lack of sleep); snoring (including sleep apnea); parasomnias (sleep walking, teeth grinding or bruxism, restless legs); medical illness (Alzheimer's disease, benign prostatic hypertrophy, menopause); emotional problems (depression, stress); and environmental sleep disturbance.

Where there is a serious sleep problem, medical help should be sought.

For many, abstaining from the evening cup of coffee may help improve sleep. Also, refraining from ingesting other methylxanthines such as tea, chocolate, and soft drinks will likely help as well.

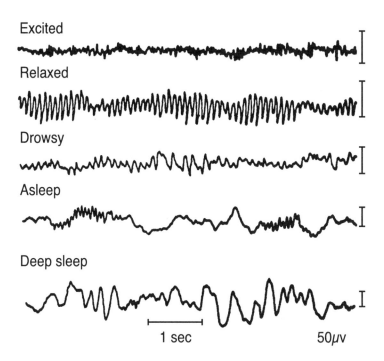

Excited

Relaxed

Drowsy

Asleep

Deep sleep

1 sec   50μv

Electro encephalogram (EEG) records of electrical brain activity in humans.

In addition to common sense remedies, one of the best ways of recapturing normal sleep patterns lies with HGH. Because poor sleep may drastically alter our production of HGH, restoring our levels of HGH can help break this cycle. Restoration of HGH levels has been shown to bring back the normal sleep patterns we had in our younger days. Not only does it restore deep sleep, it restores REM sleep. Quoting Dr. Chein: "...amazingly, although HGH treatment increased REM sleep time by 27 minutes, the total sleep time needed by patients was decreased. With this came a significantly improved sense of well being, and an increase in daytime energy."

[Dr. White and Dr. McLeod are presently involved in a clinical trial with various sleep agents to determine which maximizes deep sleep, and thus HGH release at night.]

Energy

Without energy there would be nothing happening - no motion, no warmth, no life. For all living things, including human beings, it is energy that is an essential animating force. Without it we become inert, inanimate.

Dr. Bengtssön has observed that the near universal symptom he has seen in HGH deficient patients is their lifeless, low energy state. With HGH therapy, most of these patients came out of this "zombie" state, and returned to something approximating normal.

In their study at Palm Springs, Dr. Chein and Dr. Terry found a whopping 84% of patients who reported an improvement in energy levels after HGH treatment. In that same study, 78% reported an improvement in their attitude toward life.

This last figure should not surprise us. When our health is improving, when we are sleeping like we did a decade or two earlier, and when we are feeling energetic and renewed, we are bound to experience an improved attitude toward life. Because when you add up all the improvements that HGH can make in you, the bottom line is: you feel good.

Effective Growth Hormone Administration
(Low Dose, High Frequency) in 202 Patients.

L. Cass Terry, M.D., Ph.D. and Edmund Chein, M.D.
Medical College of Wisconsin and
Palm Springs Life Extension Institute

Energy, Emotions & Memory	% of patients showing improvement
Energy Level	**84%**
Emotional Stability	**67%**
Attitude Toward Life	**78%**
Memory	**62%**

Assessment Study Conducted

Feeling Good

Some of you now in your 40's, and many in your 50's, will be able to recall seeing James Brown on TV doing his signature song "I Feel Good". It was a unique performance, bursting with life and energy. You could not get more life and energy from a jumping bean doing the jitterbug. While he did the song - not just sang it but "did" it - he was in total animation: dancing and twirling, jumping and spinning. If you tied a jar of cream to his hands or feet, you'd have butter in no time.

When James Brown did "I Feel Good" you knew that he did, indeed, feel good. You simply could not imagine anyone ever feeling better than that. Years later a song came out entitled "I Feel Better Than James Brown". You knew at once that the intent was total irony, because how could anyone feel better than James Brown?

And yet that is how we would all like to feel - if not

better than James Brown, then at least to feel good. And that is what HGH can do for us. It can make us feel good!

We can look at all the studies and statistics on HGH, all the charts and graphs, but in the end what matters most is how it makes us feel.

Of course, we want this good feeling to be ongoing and long lasting, not transitory and ephemeral, as is the case for most remedies and potions. We don't want it leaving us with some sort of hangover, as is the case for alcohol. We don't want harmful side effects, as is the case for some prescription drugs. And in each of these cases, HGH comes through with flying colors. This is especially so with the use of secretogogues, where HGH levels are restored to optimal levels, and not beyond.

HGH makes us feel good because it makes us healthy. It makes us feel good because it makes our physiology younger, the way it was ten or twenty years before. It rejuvenates our cells, tissues, and organs. We feel good because we've lost fat and we've gained muscle. We've lost wrinkles, the face looks younger. We've lost many of the aches and pains, and we sleep better now, like we did when we were young. As for sex, we're as peppy as a preppie. And we've got the renewed energy to go with it - maybe not like James Brown, but we're getting there. So why wouldn't we feel good?

And although we might take satisfaction in knowing that these improvements all come from the effects of HGH rejuvenating our tissues and organs, and that inside our bodies we are turning back the clock, the ultimate payoff is simply that we feel good. We feel good. Almost as good as James Brown. And tomorrow is going to be even better. So look out, Tin Pan Alley!

As the incredible Canadian Rock Legend, Bobby Curtola, sings: HGH may be just like his gold record song "The Real Thing". For human beings at this point in anti-aging research, there is nothing better than the hormonal power of HGH to reverse the ravages of time, and as Dr. Klatz notes in his book, *Grow Young with HGH*, "some of the best HGH releasers were the amino acids. These, in combination with a dietary program and exercise, can offer results which are very significant."

Spring Morn, Spring Mourn

As if from a dream you awaken. As if from a mist you arise. You move to an open window where curtains are billowing softly in the breeze. You look out the window upon a sunlit spring morning, trees and meadows in the distance, and in the courtyard below, standing in the streaming sun you see...yourself.

It is a younger you - you as you were ten or fifteen years ago - trim, muscled, almost athletic looking. The skin on your face is taut and tanned, your smile beams, filled with the joy of simply being young.

And you remember those days, and how it was, and how you were, and how good it all was. So good that to see yourself like that again almost hurts.

And then a wind comes up, swirling leaves into the air that were left from last autumn, taking them round and round, higher and higher. And then the wind eases and the leaves begin floating down. And now the courtyard is empty and you are gone, and there are only a few scattered leaves slowly drifting down through the air. And peer as you may through the window, that person below is gone, that younger person you once were is gone...and as you look off over the fields there are no words in you, just a feeling, a deep poignant pang inside you that says...if only...

To Date, HGH is the Best Bet in Preventing the "if Only" Syndrome.

SECTION: IV

Other Hormones

"Total hormone replacement therapy is like assembling all the sections of an orchestra...and in order to play the music of a beautiful symphony, you need every instrument from the tuba to the triangle."

– Dr. Edmund Chein

"Remember, we only want to replace hormones to their optimal levels, and not beyond. In order to replace all the hormones effectively, you need a doctor's involvement."

– Dr. Edmund Chein

"GH study from Johns Hopkins University showed the benefits of balancing hormones that decline with age."

– The Harman /Blackman

"Long term GH replacement is safe and beneficial. It improves cardiac performance and increases bone density."

– Ter Matten J.- JCEM '99

"No evidence that GH replacement therapy affects the risk of cancer or cardiovascular disease."

– Vance et al,

New England Journal of Medicine
October '99

Other Hormones

OPTIMAL LEVELS, WORKING IN HARMONY

There are many other hormones in the body besides HGH. And although the scope of the function of most is usually quite narrow when compared to that of HGH, each of them does play an important and necessary part in the overall health of the body.

Just as tradesmen such as plumbers or electricians play a specific but necessary role in the maintenance of a large building, so too it is for the roles played by hormones such as estrogen or testosterone. All of these hormones play their own particular and necessary role in maintaining the entire body in good health.

We saw earlier that the levels of HGH in the body tend to decline with age. This is also the case for many other hormones in the body. They, too, tend to decline with age.

To keep the body healthy and fit, it is desirable to have all the hormones working at optimal levels. That allows them to carry on their work in harmony with one another. If one hormone is working at a low level, it can interfere with the performance of others.

ROAD TO LONGEVITY, DOCTERS' SECRETS

Major Hormone Pathways

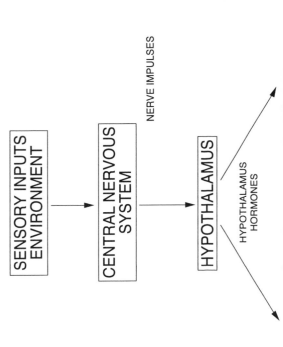

SENSORY INPUTS ENVIRONMENT

CENTRAL NERVOUS SYSTEM

NERVE IMPULSES

HYPOTHALAMUS

HYPOTHALAMUS HORMONES

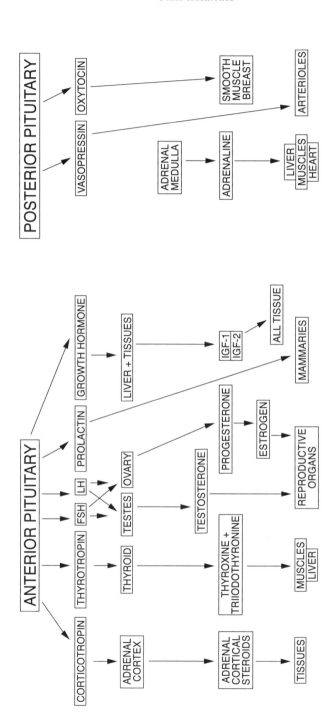

In our analogy of the tradesmen doing building maintenance, we can readily see that if the plumbers are short in manpower and have to rush their work they, will likely do shoddy work. And in rushing, if they have left pipes in place that are leaking water onto the electrical wires, this will interfere with work the electricians are doing. To say the least. Conversely, if the electricians are short in manpower and in trying to make do, leave bare wires in contact with water pipes, they jeopardize the work of the plumbers. Another grave understatement.

And so it is for the hormones in the body. The body is designed to have the hormones work with one another in a grand harmony. When one is not at an optimal level, others may suffer in their performance, even to where their levels in the body are diminished.

We have seen that HGH, working throughout the body to confer a more youthful physiology, is often capable of assisting in the elevation of other hormonal levels in the body. However, in cases of serious hormone depletion, and where more intensive measures are needed, the replacement of a specific hormone - and even more than one - may be indicated.

When used appropriately, under medical supervision, the effects of hormone replacement therapy will be comparable to that of increasing the number of plumbers or electricians doing maintenance work in the building - it will supply enough of them to do the job properly. With sufficient numbers of tradesmen, water pipes will not be left leaking but will be repaired; electrical wires will not be left bare but will be taped over or replaced. Similarly, with sufficient levels of all the hormones in operation, the otherwise healthy body will function as it should, without problems.

Unlike HGH, whose levels can be raised safely through the use of secretogogues (without danger of the level being raised unnaturally high), these other hormones should be used only under strict medical super-

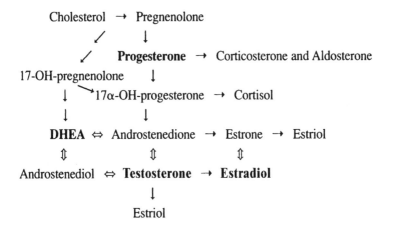

Metabolic pathway of steroid hormones.

vision. The intent of *replacement* therapy is replacement - not in raising the levels higher than normal to achieve some superhuman effect.

The desired objective is to achieve optimal levels for all hormones, to have them working in balance and harmony, not to artificially jack up this one or that one, as has unfortunately been the case with some "athletes". The objective of attaining ideal levels will be best achieved under the close supervision of a medical doctor. To prevent unwise self medication, a number of these hormones are available only by prescription.

Estrogen

We will begin our survey of the major hormones that have been used in hormone replacement therapy with the sex steroid, estrogen. For one thing, most readers will have heard something of estrogen replacement therapy, and its astounding benefits. For another, estrogen, in particular, points up the need for caution in employing replacement therapy. Much of what we have learned concerning the need for balanced levels of all the

Estradiol

hormones working together, has come about from early work with estrogen. For example, it was found that to achieve success in eliminating problems involving the menstrual cycle - especially mood swings - it was necessary to achieve suitable levels of both estrogen and another hormone, progesterone. Also, since estrogen replacement alone has been linked to some cancers, especially uterine cancer, the use of estrogen here again points up the need for caution.

Estrogen is a female hormone, but levels occur in males as well. Its role in women is largely concerned with their development from girlhood onward, and in the maintenance of female traits and characteristics, as well as regulating their cycles of ovulation. Estrogen is produced mainly in the adrenal glands and the ovaries, and the levels of estrogen are under the control of the pituitary gland. It is derived from cholesterol via its precursor, pregnenolone, which is produced in the mitochondria of the cells.

In humans the main types of estrogen are estriol, estradiol, and estrone. These estrogens are each quite different and for this reason are used differently in therapeutics. For osteoporosis, estradiol has the greatest effect. However, this estrogen has the maximum effect

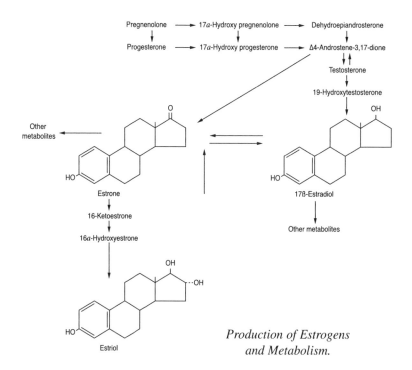

Production of Estrogens and Metabolism.

on breast estrogen receptors. Estradiol has 1000 times the affinity for breast receptors over estriol, and for this reason it is avoided if possible in women with painful breasts, or with a high risk of cancer. Estrone is easily converted to Estradiol, so the dangers for estrone are the same. We use estriol as the safest effective estrogen for the vagina and vulva, when there is a deficiency here causing symptoms like dryness. There has been controversy about estrone derivatives having an important role in breast cancer and also in prostate cancer. Estrogens are different from the other hormones because they have a phenolated A-ring that attaches to the estrogen receptor site on the cells. The great problem that we face now is that many of the sprays and plastics also contain this structure and will be dangerously active on humans as non-biodegrading xenoestrogens. Many meats and dairy products may have potent xenoestrogens that are potentially even more stimulating to the estrogen receptor than are the natural estrogens. There may be a feminization happening right now that is resulting from petrochemicals in our environment that will decrease male fertility and increase the risks for certain cancers.

One of estrogen's main functions is to control sexual development, a process in which estrogen plays a central role. A few years before menarche (the time at which a girl experiences her first menstrual period) estrogen levels begin to rise. Around the age of twelve or thirteen they are high enough to bring about ovulation. Somewhat earlier than this, a girl begins developing breasts, and secondary sex characteristics such as underarm and pubic hair. Estrogen levels then fluctuate monthly in producing the menstrual cycle and then, some years before menopause, estrogen levels begin to fall.

Not infrequently, during the years of fertility, the menstrual cycle may bring its own problems, especially as a woman reaches her thirties and beyond. Symptoms such as severe cramps, are not uncommon, as well as intense mood swings, the latter often coming under the general heading of PMS (premenstrual syndrome). We have seen that adjusting the levels of estrogen and progesterone - in proper balance - has been effective in curtailing these symptoms.

Not infrequently, PMS may in fact be due to an excess of estrogens and to a deficiency of progesterone. Estrogen dominance or estrogen excess may be associated with the following:

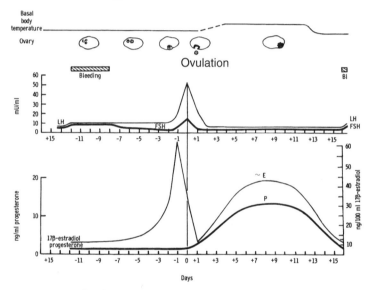

Blood Hormone Levels with Menstrual Cycle.
(Bleeding = Menses)

1. Breast pain and swelling.

2. Blood sugar abnormalities.

3. Body fat increase.

4. Water retention and bloating.

5. Cancer of the uterus and breast.

6. Thyroid dysfunction.

7. Depression, irritability, and fatigue.

8. Headaches and worsened migraines.

9. Infertility, miscarriages, and menstrual irregularities.

10. Memory loss and unclear thinking.

11. Phlebitis and blood clotting problems.

12. Decreased sex drive.

For most women, the estrogen levels will begin falling as she goes through her thirties. With the approach of menopause, some women will begin experiencing dry skin, brittle hair, and a loss of libido. Finally, as menopause itself arrives, many women will experience hot flashes, depression, loss of energy and even crying spells. For many women, estrogen replacement has shown that it can manage and reduce these symptoms. Some studies have shown a small increase in the rate of breast cancer for women taking mostly synthetic estrogens, but the interesting point is that the cancers that develop while patients are taking estrogens are of a better grade or are better differentiated, allowing for better treatment chances than those developing breast cancer while not on Hormone Replacement Therapy (HRT).

Besides falling estrogen levels, a large factor in these menopausal symptoms appears to lie with falling progesterone levels, which we will deal with shortly. Progesterone levels fall dramatically before menopause and as Dr. Jerilynn Prior points out, dropping levels of estrogen do not explain the symptoms of menopause. Western women tend to have higher estrogen levels than their eastern counterparts, likely due to diet that promotes obesity. With increased levels of an enzyme called aromatase found in fat cells that convert testosterone into estradiol, we would expect chubby men to have breast tissue and less body hair than thin athletic men. Since many women around the world do not experience the severe menopausal symptoms that western women do, the dramatic changes from such high levels of estrogen in the west may be the responsible factor.

Estrogen therapy can benefit women after menopause. Several studies looking at the benefits of estrogen and synthetic progestins have been done. The results have shown positive effects by raising HDL good cholesterol, but have also shown raised levels of triglycerides (blood fats) seen in the

Ethinyl estradiol

Diethylstilbestrol

Some synthetic Estrogens.
(Compare with natural Estradiol)

Postmenopausal Estrogen/Progestin Interventions (PEPI Trial) 1995 and Nurses' Health Study 1996. Also the Heart and Estrogen/Progestin Replacement Study (HERS) 1998 showed that women with pre-existent heart disease (50 % of women in their 50's) had 1.5 times the number of cardiac events in the first year of Hormone Replacement Therapy (HRT). The moral of the study may be that beginning HRT at the first signs of menopause may be important, and that such therapy should not be deferred for too many years. There may also be a subset of women that are predisposed to problems with estrogen that will be identified in the future. The Women's Health Initiative (WHI) is now under way and will answer some of our questions about the advantages of HRT for cardiovascular health in different groups of women.

The benefits of estrogen replacement therapy are as follows:

1. Improved longevity.

2. Relief from fatigue, sweating, hot flushing.

3. Relief from depression.

4. Loss of wrinkles and dry skin.

5. Improved libido and energy levels.

6. Diminished osteoporosis (possibly with estrogen stimulating HGH production).

7. Decreased atherosclerosis (less LDL, more HDL cholesterol).

8. Less heart attack, stroke, heart failure, if taken before disease starts.

9. Improved brain function with protection from Alzheimer's disease.

10. Proper menstrual cycles and fertility.

Results published in 1996 from the Kaiser Permanente study done in California showed that the death rate from all causes was reduced by 44% in post menopausal women who were on estrogen replacement.

However, since estrogen therapy has been linked to an increased risk of endometrial cancer in women, caution

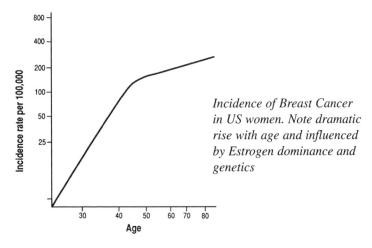

Incidence of Breast Cancer in US women. Note dramatic rise with age and influenced by Estrogen dominance and genetics

is the watchword. And balance. Research has shown that when progesterone is administered along with estrogen, the chance of developing uterine (endometrial) cancer is greatly reduced.

Recently, it has been shown that the risk of developing breast cancer with hormone replacement therapy together is unlikely to be increased. The beneficial effects of natural estrogens may be negated by certain un-natural progestins. The goal should be to bring the hormonal levels back, in balance, to what is near normal, and this should be carried out under the auspices of a medical doctor who can monitor the levels of these potentially life saving hormones.

Progesterone

Progesterone is another important female hormone. We have seen that it works in close conjunction with estrogen.

Produced in the corpus luteum (the follicle that ruptures during ovulation), the adrenal glands, and in the placenta during pregnancy, progesterone plays a crucial role in a woman's menstrual cycle. It is instrumental in bringing about changes in the uterus, changes which prepares the uterus lining for the reception of a fertilized egg. Where fertilization does not occur, the progesterone levels drop, causing the prepared lining of the uterus to be sloughed off.

Progesterone is largely responsible for mood swings associated with the menstrual cycle that some women are subject to. It is the low level of progesterone just prior to menstruation that is responsible for bringing on the symptoms of PMS experienced by these women. By undergoing treatment that brings both progesterone and estrogen to normal levels, many women have found relief from these pre menstrual mood swings.

As women get into their late 30's their progesterone levels decrease. As they go into menopause, these levels then tend to fluctuate wildly. These fluctuating levels of progesterone, combined with low levels of estrogen, bring on the various symptoms of menopause. By bringing the levels of both hormones into balance, and back to levels found in pre-menopausal women, these menopausal symptoms, for many women, have been reduced or eliminated.

Progesterone

If menopausal symptoms continue, with normal progesterone and estrogen levels, then many women turn to Primrose Oil, Black Cohosh (Remifemin) or clonidine (Dixarit) to control symptoms of flushing and sweats.

Another important facet of progesterone's activity is its strong involvement in a woman's sex drive.

Progesterone is the hormone thought to exercise the strongest influence in this regard - in conjunction with testosterone - and progesterone is considered to produce the heightened libido many women experience after ovulation.

One of progesterone's strongest benefits is in preventing osteoporosis. Its effects in this area are stronger still when used in conjunction with estrogen. Even on its own, progesterone has shown a significant effect in maintaining bone density. Studies conducted by Dr. John Lee and by Dr. Jerilynn Prior at the University of British Columbia have shown

Progesterone Metabolism.

that progesterone can not only stop bone destruction, but it can also stimulate the osteoblasts to form new bone.

A complete list of the benefits of natural progesterone replacement is as follows:

1. Better sleep pattern.

2. Improved libido (sex drive).

3. Better glucose tolerance.

4. Helps protect against uterine cancer, fibroids, fibrocystic breasts and maybe breast cancer.

5. Lipolytic (burns fat) and mild diuretic.

6. Elevates mood and helps diminish depression (especially postpartum).

7. Essential for proper reproduction and healthy pregnancy.

8. Reverses osteoporosis by stimulating osteoblasts.

9. Improves thyroid function.

10. Improves blood clotting pathways.

11. Decreases the chance of endometriosis.

12. Improvement in allergies and in some autoimmune disorders.

As regards the two female hormones, estrogen and progesterone, there is a further cautionary note. Some versions of these hormones have been shown to bring on more side effects than others.

For example, the estrogens obtained from the urine of pregnant mares is not totally identical with estrogen produced by humans. And although the use of these "mare" hormones by women will not have them breaking out into spontaneous whinnies, as some comedians have portrayed, they have caused some women to experience other side effects. These include excessive water retention, headaches, and moodiness.

There are also synthetic hormones produced by drug companies that are available. These designer hormones are generally not identical, at the molecular level, with those natural hormones produced in the body. Synthetic estrogen receptor modifiers (SERMS) will have a place in future treatment.

Finally, there are natural versions of both estrogen and progesterone available. These forms of the hormones are identical, at the molecular level, with those produced in the body. And in general, women taking the natural versions of either progesterone or estrogen, have tended to report fewer unpleasant side effects. We generally use natural estradiol or combinations with estriol when needed and we use Prometrium (micronized natural progesterone) or progesterone cream applied at night to various body sites. Often the natural cycle of estrogen and progesterone will be maintained to mimic premenopausal cycles and many women feel better with this approach. Saliva levels or blood levels are always followed for proper replacement techniques.

Δ4(5)-17a-Ethynyl-17-hydroxyestren-3-one
(norethindrone, Norlutin)

Δ5(10)-17a-Ethynyl-17-
hydroxyestren-3-one

6a-Methyl-17a-acetoxyprogesterone
(medroxyprogesterone, Provera)

An example of orally active Progestins (synthetics)

Again, as with any hormone replacement therapy, estrogen and progesterone therapy should be carried out only under the direct care and supervision of a medical doctor.

Testosterone

Testosterone is the principal male sex hormone. Although testosterone does also occur in women, (produced in the ovaries and adrenal glands), testosterone levels in women are only about a tenth of those in men.

In men, testosterone is produced in the testes and adrenal glands. It is the chief player in bringing about sexual development in the male. Andropause (male equivalent of the menopause) is finally gaining wide attention around the world, as demonstrated by the concern raised at the Second World Congress on the Aging Male in Geneva, February 2000, where the World Health Organization described male health as a "neglected" area of modern medicine. Dr. Richard Bebb of Vancouver, Canada reported some of the striking benefits of testosterone therapy for bone density of the spines in androgen deficient males. Dr. Alvaro Palacios from Venezuela reported oral

Testosterone

testosterone undecanoate was effective in treating men with PADAM (symptoms of physical, vasomotor, psychological and sexual problems in aging men). London cardiologist, Dr. Peter Collins, states, " it seems that testosterone acts as an anti-ischemic drug in men with coronary heart disease and decreased levels of plasma testosterone." It is known that there are more testosterone receptors in the heart muscle than in other muscles of the human. As is the case for most of the other hormones, the levels of testosterone diminish as a man ages with the levels of free testosterone (biologically active) dropping by 2 % per year after the age of 30 years.. With the decline of testosterone levels, there is generally an accompanying decline in other aspects of a man's health that are associated with testosterone. Not many years ago, testosterone was feared by the public as a bad hormone, causing aggression and symptoms of maleness. It was even a triplicate prescription in some areas of Canada under the same control category as Demerol and Morphine.

Testosterone is involved in maintaining erectile function, and in generating the male sex drive. Further, testosterone promotes the buildup of protein into muscle (anabolism), and works against protein breakdown (catabolism). Testosterone is also responsible for more calmness and assertiveness in the male, and is involved in maintaining normal male energy levels.

Although testosterone has not been studied as extensively as the female hormones, there is sufficient data to ascribe, with a high degree of probability, a number of beneficial effects to testosterone replacement therapy in males.

In looking at these beneficial effects, it might be helpful to consider, first, a condition referred to as "andropause." The concept of andropause as a male equivalent of menopause is now gaining wide acceptance in the medical establishment, particularly as it reflects a legitimate concern for male health. Longevity doctors have always been concerned with the plummeting levels of testosterone that accompany aging.

Misgivings over testosterone treatment are completely unfounded. With the proper use of this important hormone for ultimate male health, there are very few untoward side effects. On the other hand, with proper use, testosterone may prevent much illness, malaise, fatigue, apathy, and aging in the male population. The authors have rarely seen a male exhibiting robust good health while at the same time showing testosterone levels that were well below the normal range.

Researchers Heller and Myers concluded 50 years ago that there were a number of symptoms that could be identified with andropause. Some of these are as follows:

1. Mental: anxiety, irritability, insomnia, depression, antisocial , poor concentration.

2. Vasomotor: hot flashes, sweats, palpitations, headaches.

3. Constitutional: weakness, fatigue, myalgia, nausea, constipation, weight loss.

4. Urinary: frequency, hesitancy, decreased force.

5. Sexual: decreased libido, decreased pleasure, impotency.

All of the above may be reversible with testosterone replacement.

Synthesis of testicular androgen and estrogen. Heavy arrows show major pathways. Circled numbers show enzymes:

①, 20,22-desmolase (P-450); ⑥, 3ß-hydroxysteroid dehydrogenase and $\triangle^5$, $\triangle^4$-isomerase; ③, 17-hydroxylase (P-450); ⑤, 17,20-desmolase (P-450); ⑥, 17-ketoreductase; ", 5 " reductase; ', aromatase.

There are many causes of decreased production of testosterone from the testes in men or from the adrenal glands. Some of these include: drugs, radiation, alcohol, chronic obstructive pulmonary disease, renal failure, cancer, cirrhosis of the liver, hemochromatosis, chronic diseases, nutritional deficiencies, genetics, trauma, pituitary tumors, and obesity. Estrogen will fill some of the testosterone receptors in the brain, such that the hypothalamus will send a message to the testes to produce less testosterone. As we age, our production of Sex Hormone Binding Globulin (SHBG) increases possibly due to the stimulus of extra estrogens that occur. This protein actually binds the testosterone to make it unavailable for its role in stimulating receptor sites around the body. Normally only 2-3 % of the testosterone is free from attachment to proteins.

In an area crucial to males - that of sexual function - testosterone replacement has produced results that are very positive: increases in libido and sexual activity. Also, testosterone has been shown to promote increases in bone density and muscle mass, while at the same time bringing about decreases in body fat.

Dr. Eugene Shippen from PA, USA recognizes that the estrogen / free testosterone ratio is the important predictor of male well-being, and thus the method of testosterone replacement is the most important decision to be made to keep the conversion to estrogen at a minimum. If we allow the testosterone levels to peak to enormous non-physiological levels as by testosterone injections, then we are priming our patients for symptom swings, and conversions to the unwanted estrogens. We generally use methods to slowly increase the levels of testosterone in the serum. We have used Andriol in pill form, as well as the testosterone patch (Androderm or Testoderm) which will gain more popularity and we routinely supply prescriptions for testosterone cream, usually a 5% cream, with 1 cc applied each night to the armpits before bed. We never allow the cream to be applied to the scrotum for fear of conversion to dihydrotestosterone, another hormone that we will discuss.

We certainly need the effects of testosterone all over our body and not just to the testes. Levels of total testosterone and free testosterone need to be monitored as well as Estradiol levels, and if possible levels of dihydrotestosterone (DHT). This potent form of testosterone can cause central scalp baldness and can lead to benign prostatic hypertrophy (BPH). Two enzymes of 5-alpha reductase cause the conversion of testosterone to DHT, one in the skin causing sebum (skin oil) production and changing hair growth. The other 5-alpha reductase in the prostate will increase the production of DHT to allow increased fibrous and muscular size of the prostate - sometimes out of control - blocking the flow of urine because of benign prostatic hypertrophy (BPH). In our practice we liberally use saw palmetto (Serenoa repens), a herbal extract from berries to inhibit 5-alpha reductase that may also suppress estrogen.

Testosterone conversion to more potent Dihydrotestosterone (DHT) may aggravate acne and promote baldness.

We reserve the use of finasteride (Proscar and Propecia) for the major suppression of DHT when the levels are much too high or when BPH or baldness are major issues to be tackled. Before anyone is even considered for testosterone replacement, a thorough exam with digital rectal is done, and serum PSA (prostate specific antigen) is a must to detect prostate cancer. Patients with snoring and /or sleep apnea are cautioned that testosterone replacement worsens this condition and discussion with your doctor is imperative.

Prostate Cancer

The question on everyone's mind is the relationship of cancer and testosterone replacement. Once a man has the diagnosis of prostate cancer, all physicians agree that testosterone must be stopped to prevent the existing cancer cells from proliferating. This is done in cancer patients by administering leuprolide, which mimics the LH releasing hormone in the hypothalamus and cutting off the supply of luteinizing hormone (LH) to the testes, preventing testosterone production. The other method is for the cancer patient to take flutamide to block the uptake of testosterone at the receptor site. Of all studies reviewed, there still are a few that find some correlation between cancer of the prostate and testosterone or DHT levels. By far the majority of dozens of studies show absolutely that testosterone does not cause prostate cancer. There may be evidence that cancer risk may be actually reduced by keeping the ratio of testosterone / estrogen near to 40:1, as it is in a young man. Given these effects of testosterone replacement therapy, it is not hard to imagine some males - young and old - going overboard on testosterone treatments: the young attempting to become supermen; the old trying to recapture their youth, and the sexual prowess that accompanied it.

Here again it must be emphasized, the desired goal is to bring the hormone to normal, youthful levels, not beyond. For most normal young men, trying to attain higher than normal testosterone levels is unnecessary and potentially hazardous. For older men, attaining normal levels (not exceeding them), that are in balance with their other hormones, is the proper goal. It is a goal best attempted under the care of one's doctor. Going beyond normal levels on one's own is simply to prove the old adage: There's no fool like an old fool.

Although testosterone is principally a male hormone, it is found at significant levels in the female. There has been less research done on the effects of testosterone in women, but this is presently being corrected.

Meanwhile, it is known that testosterone levels tend to decrease with age in women, as is the case for the other hormones as well. Which suggests that if a woman seeks to replace her declining female hormones, she would be well advised to undertake testosterone replacement also.

It is a near certainty that testosterone, along with the female hormones, plays a significant role in the female libido. In a woman's monthly cycle, her testosterone levels, as well as her progesterone levels, are at a high point after ovulation. Which is when many women experience their strongest sexual desire.

Another indication of testosterone's link with the female hormones is seen in another area, bone formation. We saw that when progesterone was included with estrogen in replacement therapy, not only was osteoporosis retarded, but it was reversed. So too is the case when testosterone is added to estrogen in those circumstances.

As further research is completed there will, no doubt, be much more information forthcoming concerning the function of testosterone in both men and women.

DHEA

DHEA (Dehydroepiandrosterone) is a hormone that is produced in the adrenal cortex. It is a precursor to the sex hormones estrogen and testosterone. Like most other hormones in the body, the levels of DHEA diminish with age, beginning the decline at around age 30. DHEA is only produced in primates and there seems to be no obvious feedback system, so that no serious side effects have been seen with huge doses. DHEA is easily obtained in the U.S. over the counter at many stores but is only available in western Canada, from Kripp's Drugstore legally, with a prescription with special authority from Ottawa. Commercially, DHEA comes from diosgenin, a common sterol from wild yams. Generally as cortisol levels rise, DHEA levels fall, which explains the role of stress in reducing levels of this hormone. DHEA levels are highest in the morning and it is weakly bound to the protein, albumin. The metabolite, DHEA-sulfate is cleared slowly and this is what we measure with saliva or blood tests. There may be receptors for DHEA in our brain and body and DHEA seems to interact with brain neurotransmitters such as serotonin (which is affected by Prozac), but these receptors have yet to be identified

Given that the decline of DHEA levels is accompanied by a number of diseases and conditions that also tend to accompany aging, these lowering levels of DHEA have been regarded as a possible causative agent of them, or at least to being involved in their occurrence. For example, low levels of DHEA tend to be found in cases of obesity, diabetes, heart disease, cancer and immune deficiency. This suggests to some, that by raising the levels of DHEA, we might deter some of these diseases or conditions, or at the least, postpone their arrival to a point later in our lives.

*Dehydroepiandrosterone
(DHEA)*

There is considerable anecdotal evidence that DHEA is effective in promoting weight loss, and gains in muscle mass. One study involving rats showed that the rats treated with DHEA tended to accumulate less body fat than did a control group that was on the same diet. It is possible, however, that DHEA is achieving these results by controlling appetite. Quoting Dr. Chein: "Some statistics have also shown that DHEA works as an appetite suppressant."

Should this prove to be the case, there might be a concern that along with the suppressed appetite, there might also be an accompanying decrease in nutrient intake.

There is evidence that DHEA is capable of promoting a more healthy heart. One study by Elizabeth Barret-Connor at the University of San Diego, tended to support this idea. The findings of her study showed that the men who had high levels of DHEA, had half the likelihood of being subject to heart disease. Undoubtedly, more research is ongoing in this area. Studies in 1994 at the University of California, San Diego, School of Medicine, showed that middle aged subjects taking 50 mg of DHEA for 3 months had improved well being of mood, energy, sleep, and were more relaxed. Of course as the media became more involved then DHEA became the new "Fountain of Youth" and the new panacea.

Low levels of DHEA have been shown to accompany immune deficiency disease. One study showed that for people infected with HIV, there was twice the chance of developing full blown AIDS if their DHEA levels were low.

Because DHEA is a precursor to the sex hormones, it does have an effect on them. One likely consequence of being a precursor to these hormones is that it can bring about an increase in their levels. This would almost certainly account for reports and anecdotal evidence indicating that DHEA is capable of improving sexual performance and sexual pleasure.

To date, DHEA has been associated with very few negative side effects. Concerning these side effects Dr. Chein has written: "Because it is a precursor to the sex hormones, (primarily testosterone) DHEA can have androgenic (testosterone-like) effects on women, causing

Dehydroepiandrosterone sulfate
DHEA-S

Dehydroepiandrosterone
DHEA

Equilibrium of DHEA-S Production

increased facial hair, menstrual changes, and acne. Some overusers have reported mood changes and increased aggression. Some male patients experienced nasal congestion and mild insomnia. And there are also cases of enlarged prostate that we've encountered with self-prescribed, excessive DHEA users who come to the Palm Springs Life Extension Institute." We see many patients taking 25 mg / day in the a.m. on weekdays.

We constantly monitor DHEA-S levels, check prostates and watch for signs of excess androgens. All of which underscores still again the need to proceed with hormone replacement under the auspices of a doctor.

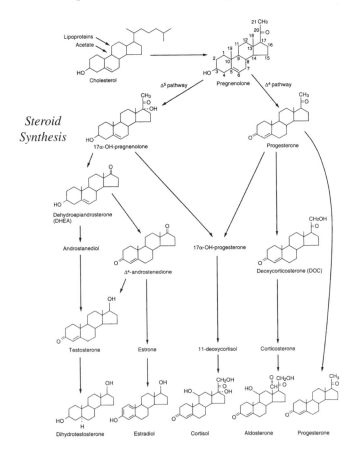

Steroid Synthesis

[Studies done by Dr. McLeod and Dr. White indicate that DHEA levels may be decreased by statin drugs administered for lowering cholesterol. Further studies are ongoing and more detailed results are expected in the near future.]

Pregnenolone

Just as DHEA is a precursor to the sex hormones, pregnenolone is a precursor to DHEA. If we look at DHEA as being the mother hormone to the sex hormones, then pregnenolone is the grandmother. It is not surprising, then, that pregnenolone, like DHEA, is produced in the brain and in the adrenal glands. And like the majority of the body's other hormones, pregnenolone levels, too, tend to decline with age.

Since pregnenolone is a mother hormone to DHEA, and grandmother to the sex hormones, it is again not surprising that raising the levels of pregnenolone tends to bring about raised levels of the other hormones as well.

Pregnenolone is found in very high concentrations in the brain. This, no doubt, is one reason why it has been looked at for its effects on brain function. Studies so far indicate that pregnenolone is indeed capable of enhancing mental performance. Some of these enhancements take the form of improved memory and improved capacity for learning. Also, pregnenolone has been shown to bring about improvements in mood and decreases in depression.

Decades back, pregnenolone was used in easing the pain of arthritis. Then, in the 1940's, cortisone came onto the scene, relegating pregnenolone to the back of the shelf. However, with serious side effects to cortisone treatment showing up, pregnenolone may well see a resurgence in this area of application.

Because pregnenolone is a precursor to DHEA, and in turn to the sex hormones, this would tend to explain why it is capable of raising the levels of these hormones. Further, since pregnenolone does affect the sex hormones, it should not surprise us that it does serve somewhat different functions in men than it does in women. In women, more of the pregnenolone goes into the production of estrogen, while in men, more of it is used to produce testosterone. (A good thing - otherwise men would sing soprano and women would grow beards.) However, with this differing role in males and females, and given the dangers of side effects where levels of DHEA, estrogen, or testosterone are brought to a point higher than are normally found in the body, one is well advised to have pregnenolone treatment done under the care of a doctor, with monitoring being done on all the hormones that may be affected by pregnenolone.

Melatonin

Melatonin has been widely touted in the news over the past few years as the latest anti-aging discovery. It has been reported as conferring numerous benefits in combating the aging process, and as well, it has been cited for its efficacy in helping to regulate the body's daily rhythms.

Melatonin

Melatonin is a hormone produced by the pineal gland, a gland tucked away inside the brain, back in behind the eyes. The pineal gland may, in fact, be what some eastern mystics have referred to as the "third eye". And because secretions of melatonin by the pineal gland are affected by light, this may not be as fanciful as it seems.

Melatonin has shown that it strongly affects the body's circadian, or daily rhythms. As daylight fades through the evening hours, the levels of melatonin begin to rise, reaching their peak around midnight. As these levels rise through the evening we eventually begin to feel sleepy, and are ready for bed. Conversely, as dawn breaks, the levels of melatonin, which have been diminishing during the night, drop off more sharply, inducing us to awaken for the day.

Because increased levels of melatonin are conducive to sleep, it has been used in this regard, in place of a sleeping pill. So far, melatonin has shown that taken a little before bedtime, it can significantly improve sleep. In contrast with other potions and sleeping pills, melatonin has not demonstrated the kinds of side effects these other medications all too often bring on. As an added plus, melatonin has not shown itself to interfere with REM sleep. Melatonin is found to be one of the safest of hypnotics (sleeping medicines) in Children's Hospital in Vancouver, Canada.

Given melatonin's ability in regulating our circadian rhythms, it has also been used to reduce the effects of jet lag. When we fly across several time zones (e.g. New York to London), within a few hours the body is thrust into an entirely different time of day. It is put on a very different clock. In its normal physiological schedule, the body may be ready for dinner and then an evening of activity afterwards, whereas in the new time zone it is already bedtime. And around the time the body is preparing itself for a good sleep, morning has arrived and we must be about our daily activities.

Production and Metobolism of Melatonin

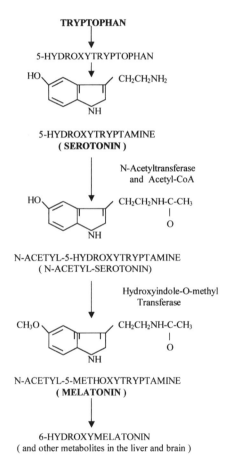

TRYPTOPHAN

5-HYDROXYTRYPTOPHAN

5-HYDROXYTRYPTAMINE
(**SEROTONIN**)

N-Acetyltransferase
and Acetyl-CoA

N-ACETYL-5-HYDROXYTRYPTAMINE
(N-ACETYL-SEROTONIN)

Hydroxyindole-O-methyl
Transferase

N-ACETYL-5-METHOXYTRYPTAMINE
(**MELATONIN**)

6-HYDROXYMELATONIN
(and other metabolites in the liver and brain)

Because melatonin levels rise towards bedtime and thereby help induce sleep, taken at the appropriate time in a new time zone, melatonin can help the body to get to sleep more readily at the new bedtime. It helps the body reset the physiological clock, so to speak. It helps the body to adjust its daily rhythms to coincide with the newly imposed external time.

Something akin to the manner of HGH, melatonin, too, can produce its effects throughout the body. Also, as is the case for most hormones, the levels of melatonin diminish as we age. Around age 45 these levels drop off sharply, and it has been posited that it is these decreasing levels of melatonin that are at least partly responsible for the levels of other hormones beginning their age-related decline.

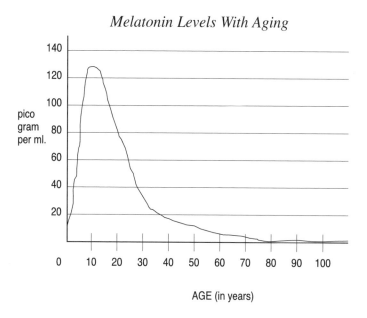

Melatonin Levels With Aging

AGE (in years)

Research conducted by Dr. Walter Pierpaoli and Dr. William Regelson demonstrated rather dramatically the involvement of melatonin in the aging process. They transferred the pineal glands of young mice into old mice, and those of the old mice into the young mice. The old mice with the young pineal glands showed a rejuvenation on many fronts: renewed vigor and energy, youthful looking fur, younger skin. Most significantly, they lived

30% longer than normal, and maintained their youthful characteristics almost until they died.

The young mice, on the other hand, the ones whose original pineal glands had been replaced with old pineal glands, died 30% sooner than did those in the control group. They also showed a more rapid deterioration in the condition of their fur, as well as in their energy levels and vitality.

Another significant result of these experiments was that the youthful pineal gland in the old mice brought about a rejuvenation to the thymus gland. This almost certainly was a causative feature of melatonin's strong positive effect on the immune system. The thymus, we will recall, plays a crucial role in T-cell formation, serving to "incubate" the T-cells and bring them to maturity.

Another study showed that partial sleep deprivation brought about lower melatonin levels, which in turn, brought about reduced activity in the NK (natural killer) cells. The NK cells are the part of the body's army that combats viruses, and most importantly, cancer.

Melatonin has also shown itself to be a very effective antioxidant. Because it can work inside the cell, melatonin is able not only to neutralize free radicals trying to eat holes through the cell's wall, but it can even counter free radicals in the nucleus that are damaging and degrading the cell's DNA.

Although melatonin has shown a minimum of harmful side effects, there are concerns that we would be well advised to keep in mind. A cautionary note from Dr. Chein: "In studies using varying doses of melatonin, the only reported side effects included: high-dose-induced headaches, nausea, chronic grogginess, and nightmares.

Despite this apparent safety, self-prescribed melatonin users still experience some problems.

One of the main problems lies with the over-the-counter varieties of the supplement. Because melatonin is not a regulated substance, almost anyone who wants to, can manufacture it. Some formulations may be poor quality and not completely pure. This increases your risk of experiencing the side effects mentioned above, and some people have reported another problem - that the effect of melatonin wears off suddenly."

Further, to date there are no long term studies on humans that conclusively demonstrate the benefits of melatonin.

Thyroid Hormone

The thyroid gland, mainly through the secretion of thyroid hormone, has a wide ranging effect on the entire body. The gland itself takes the shape of a butterfly, and is found at the front of the trachea (windpipe), just below the larynx. The reason that thyroid hormone can affect so much of the body is that it is primarily responsible for regulating the body's metabolism. It controls the furnace, so to speak.

Hormone	Common Name	Biologic Activity
L-3,5,3',5'-Tetraiodothyronine	L-Thyroxine; T_4	100
L-3,5,3',-Triiodothyronine	T_3	300-800

T4 and T3 from Thyroid Gland

Thyroid hormone regulates the rate at which the body carries out its physiological functions, particularly in the area of fat and carbohydrate metabolism. The thyroid gland and thyroid hormone are bound up in a feedback loop that ultimately begins with the hypothalamus. We have seen how the hypothalamus was involved with the pituitary gland and levels of HGH, and a similar feedback loop occurs in the case of thyroid hormone as well. When the hypothalamus detects that the levels of thyroid hormone in the body are low, it releases thyroid releasing hormone (TRH). Thyroid releasing hormone directs the pituitary gland to secrete thyroid stimulating hormone (TSH), which in turn directs the thyroid gland to secrete thyroid hormone. As the biologically active thyroid hormone, triiodothyronine, is disseminated throughout the body, it stimulates the cells to proceed with the production of energy by means of burning fats and carbohydrates. As the thyroid hormone does its job it becomes depleted. When levels drop off sufficiently, this is detected by the hypothalamus and the cycle begins all over again.

The feedback loop we have just considered is, of course, an extreme oversimplification. We have already seen that the HGH feedback loop also affects levels of thyroid hormone (and others), and that many of the hormones affect each other, as well, in the manner of a complex Rube Goldberg machine. (Those of a certain age will recall the cartoonist's work, which invariably depicted an intricate set of contraptions wherein the initial one would set off the part it was hooked up to, and that one would in turn set off the next , and so on, until some final event was triggered.)

When levels of thyroid hormone are persistently low - a condition referred to as hypothyroidism - it is akin to

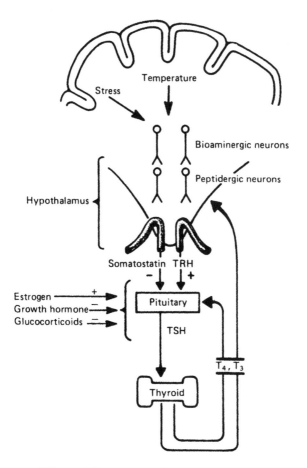

*Effects of Hormones and stress on Thyroid
production of T4 & T3.*

having the thermostat on a furnace set too low. In that circumstance, the fuel is not being burned at a normal or sufficient rate, and there is not sufficient energy or heat being produced. The building is not being kept warm enough. Checking one's temperature routinely may indicate whether the thyroid is functioning properly.

In a corresponding fashion, where people do not produce sufficient thyroid hormone to keep the metabolism of fats and carbohydrates burning at a normal rate, they too, will not be generating enough energy or heat. Often they, too, will feel cold. And much of the time they will feel fatigued and weak. Also, because they are not burning carbohydrates and fats at a normal rate, they will find themselves gaining weight in the form of stored fat.

Since the thyroid affects the body's metabolism as a whole, it also has a depressing effect on the production of certain necessary proteins, further weakening the body.

Where there is insufficient production of thyroid hormone, there is very often an accompanying weakening of the immune system. Which is why people with low levels of thyroid hormone are much more susceptible to colds, flu, and other viruses.

A number of other symptoms may accompany hypothyroidism, including a slower heart rate, high cholesterol levels, dry skin, a tendency to cramp, headaches, and infertility and menstrual difficulties in women.

Because many of the symptoms of hypothyroidism are similar to those that occur in the aging process, thyroid deficiencies sometimes go overlooked. We have seen that HGH has a singular effect on the levels of thyroid hormone, and that by increasing our levels of HGH we may also bring about increased levels of thyroid hormone as well. However, more pronounced thyroid hormone deficiencies are best corrected with thyroid hormone replacement therapy. Treatment with thyroid hormone has shown itself to be highly effective in bringing the body's metabolism back into normal limits, and thereby reducing or limiting the above mentioned symptoms. This is especially so in regard to restoring normal body temperature, energy levels, and weight control. All such replacement therapy, however, should be monitored and carried out under the care of a medical doctor.

Somapause

A very interesting concept is being developed embodying the idea that decreasing hormone production leads to a condition that has a specific set of symptoms that may be labeled as "somapause" or "somatopause". This term refers to a condition where many of the body's hormones are decreasing with age, especially HGH.

We have seen that, for a number of the body's hormones, the levels in the body tend to decrease with age. In the case of the sex steroids, estrogen and progesterone, this produces in women a set of conditions which are formally recognized as menopause. In men, an equivalent condition - andropause - also manifests itself (although more gradually) as the production of testosterone biologically available decreases with age. And so it is for most of the hormones we have mentioned so far, with the exception of insulin and cortisol, which often tend to increase with age, bringing their own related disease problems.

In the case of HGH, where adults exhibit low serum IGF-1 levels, a condition called Growth Hormone Deficiency Syndrome is now recognized and accepted. Some of the symptoms include impaired psychological well being, increased abdominal obesity, and reduced strength and exercise capacity. Other signs that may be indicative of growth hormone deficiency (GHD) are mixed obesity; increased hip-waist ratio; thin, dry, cool peripheral limbs; hyperlipidemia; decreased creatinine clearance; reduced lean muscle mass; reduced basal metabolic rate; fatigue; and reduced bone density. All patients with GHD should be eligible for methods to increase HGH, whether it is by use of secretogogues or by direct HGH injection.

Further, in the near future, it would appear likely that, just as menopause and andropause are formally recognized as treatable medical conditions, so too, somapause will be similarly recognized. Given that circumstance, it would appear likely, then, that somapause will become eligible for medical treatment as well.

SECTION V

Antioxidants, Minerals and Other Supplements

"It is better to wear out than to rust out."

– George Whitefield
(lived 56 years)

"When a man dies, he does not just die of the disease he has: he dies of his whole life."

– Charles Pequy

Antioxidants, Minerals and Other Supplements

FREE RADICALS

We looked at free radicals earlier and we saw that they are able to cause a great deal of harm to the cells of the body. Free radicals eat away at the cell wall, they eat away at other parts of the cell, and they eat away at the DNA in the nucleus.

If you have ever put too much bleach in your wash, and afterwards saw the deterioration and holes this produced in a T-shirt or blouse, you will have some idea of what the oxidation caused by free radicals do to the cells of the body. For many men, who may have never done a load of wash (although the bleach accident may have happened to more men than women), perhaps a different analogy might serve. If you have ever used too much fertilizer on the lawn, and applied it unevenly, you will have seen the burned out dead patches where the fertilizer has eaten away at the individual grass plants. These burned out patches in the lawn might also be likened to the effects free radicals have on our cells, tissues, and organs.

Free radicals generally consist of oxygen in one form or another, or oxygen in combination with other atoms. These free radicals all have an unpaired electron, leaving them electronically charged or unbalanced. Because of its electrical imbalance, a free radical strives to attain neutrality by trying to combine with other atoms it comes in contact with. In so doing the free radical ends up tearing atoms and molecules out of the cell wall, out of the mitochondria (impairing ATP production), even out of the DNA in the cell nucleus (affecting code or cross-links). Free radicals also attack lysosomes, and by combining with blood and tissue lipids (H_2O_2 + cholesterol), produce plaque. Sometimes the action of a free radical can rip out a molecular bit from a cell and thereby set in motion a chain reaction that creates still more free radicals drifting around wreaking havoc.

There are varying kinds of free radicals, which allows some of them to "specialize" in their own particular areas of pillage. The most important free radicals include:

- Superoxide anion radical

- Singlet oxygen

- Oxidized protein

- Organic or fatty acid hydro peroxide

- Hydroxyl radical

- Hydrogen peroxide (H_2O_2)

As we look at substances that can counter these wreckers, we will see that some of them, too, have their own areas of specialization, areas where they are especially good at knocking out particular kinds of free radicals. One of the few books explaining this subject in depth is *Doctors' Secrets: The Antioxidant Highway.*

Antioxidants

Antioxidants are substances that have the capability of countering and neutralizing free radicals, rendering them harmless. If you look at the electrical imbalance on a free radical as a short, sharp blade which it uses to hack and slice off bits of the cell which it impales on the blade, then you might look at an antioxidant as being a cork. This cork is of such a nature that it seeks out free radicals and presses itself onto the free radical's knife blade. This covers the sharp blade and prevents it from slicing and hacking any further.

We saw earlier that we can never be entirely free of free radicals. They are an integral part of our physiology, an end product of the biochemical reactions involved in our energy production. If we do physical exercise, we generate energy. In addition, we also generate free radicals. If we increase the exercise, besides the increased benefits we obtain, we also generate still more free radicals. However, we need a certain amount of exercise, so the answer is not to become sedentary and immobilized.

In addition to generating free radicals through our normal physiological processes, the modern world induces a higher level of free radicals in many of us indirectly, through the pollution and smog in the environment, through the action of the sun's radiation on our skin, through unhealthy diets, through cigarette smoke, stress, and even lack of exercise, cancer may be the result.

The obvious solution to the problem of free radicals is to reduce them wherever and however we can. We can try and exercise and spend time where the air is clean, not on a street with miles of cars belching exhaust. We can

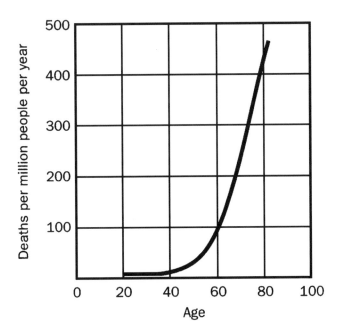

Deaths from Colon Cancer. Note dramatic rise with age.

limit our exposure to the sun. We can improve our diets. We can cut out smoking and we can try to manage our stress.

Most importantly, *we can increase the levels of antioxidants in our bodies.* We feel that this is esspecially important for glutathione, superoxide dismutase and catalase as free radical quenchers.

Increasing our intake of antioxidants is especially crucial in cases where other factors conducive to free radical formation cannot be eliminated. For instance, if we cannot escape the pollution around us, or cannot quit smoking, then it is that much more important to increase our intake of antioxidants.

High Octane Antioxidants

There are a number of substances that have demonstrated antioxidant properties that are especially strong. These are the "high octane" antioxidants. Just as a high octane fuel keeps a car engine running cleaner and more smoothly, so too these "high octane" antioxidants keep the body running cleaner and more smoothly.

The antioxidants that we will look at shortly are the best at neutralizing free radicals. In some cases, the antioxidant will neutralize them directly, while the free radicals are engaged in their vandalism. In other cases, the antioxidant will do its work by inhibiting the free radicals even before they get started. Where an antioxidant reacts with a free radical directly, it is often instrumental in halting the ensuing chain reaction, in which more and still more free radicals would have been created.

Antioxidant Vitamins

The vitamins we will look at here have been known to scientists for many decades and more, not for their role as antioxidants, but for the benefits they conferred in other aspects of human health. In a sense, some of them were discovered by their absence. For example, where early mariners came down with scurvy, it was eventually found to be caused by the absence of a previously unknown nutrient. This nutrient came to be known as vitamin C.

In the past two or three decades, however, vitamins A, C, and E have come to prominence, as well, for their properties as powerful antioxidants.

Vitamin A

Like the other vitamins, vitamin A first became of interest because it was found to be a necessary component of our diet. Vitamin A is involved in promoting heart health, a vigorous immune system, and in preventing some cancers. It is instrumental in maintaining strong bones, and healthy skin and hair. It is most necessary in maintaining good vision - night vision in particular. Vitamin A, and beta-carotene (which we will look at in a moment) are both found in carrots. Many readers - of a certain vintage - will no doubt recall the admonitions of their mothers: "Eat your carrots or you'll end up wearing glasses." Or: "You don't see rabbits wearing glasses."

Besides its nutritional benefits, vitamin A is also recognized as an excellent antioxidant. It excels at combating a form of free radical called singlet oxygen. With vitamin A we can, however, get too much of a good thing. In such cases, where there has been a much higher than normal intake of vitamin A, health problems may occur. These may include hair loss, blurred vision, nausea, fatigue, and so on. Because of this, many people will increase their intake of beta-carotene to do battle as an antioxidant in place of vitamin A, since beta-carotene is a precursor of vitamin A.

Beta-carotene

Beta-carotene can be converted into vitamin A by the body. In contrast to vitamin A, beta-carotene carries no risk when ingested in higher than normal amounts. Like vitamin A, beta-carotene helps diminish the risk of heart disease and cancer.

In addition to its traditional role in the diet beta-carotene is a powerful antioxidant.   It is especially effective in neutralizing or quenching free radicals occurring in the form of singlet oxygen, and in the form of polyunsaturated fatty-acid radicals.   Because beta-carotene is effective in areas of low oxygen concentrations (e.g. in the capillaries), and is relatively unaffected by contacts with cancer causing substances, this makes beta-carotene a super-strong warrior in the battle against free radicals.

Since most people do not get adequate amounts of beta-carotene in their diets, and since beta-carotene is very safe even when ingested in high amounts, supplements of beta-carotene are highly recommended *except for cigarette smokers* (ATBC and CARET studies).

Vitamin C

Vitamin C has been known about for a very long time.   Back in the days of the sailing ships, British mariners, after lengthy voyages at sea and living on meager, limited foodstuffs, often came down with scurvy. It was discovered that if they supplemented their diet with limes they prevented scurvy from occurring. This is how the British came to be known as "Limeys".

The matter was later explained by scientists, who found that scurvy - and a number of other conditions - was the result of a vitamin C deficiency. Since limes (and other citrus fruits) are rich in vitamin C, it was actually the inclusion of vitamin C in the limes that kept the sailors free from scurvy.

Today, vitamin C is known to be employed by the body in countless ways. It is instrumental in the production of collagen, and therefore in maintaining healthy skin. Vitamin C also helps maintain healthy bones, and teeth. It assists the body in absorbing iron more efficiently.

One of the most important functions of vitamin C in the body is as an antioxidant. Vitamin C is particularly effective in countering superoxide anion radicals and hydroxyl radicals.

Since vitamin C is water soluble, the body is not able to store it in quantity. It is best, therefore, taken daily, or if possible, two or three times a day, in smaller amounts.

Formerly, huge quantities of vitamin C were recommended by some. Today, however, because vitamin C can bring on disturbances to the digestive tract when used in large amounts, and to prevent a paradoxical oxidant effect via a so called Fenton Reaction, only about 1000 mg. per day are recommended orally. Dosages of this magnitude have recently been found effective for high blood pressure (hypertension). (Linus Pauling Institute, 2000). Given intravenously though, huge doses are effective as an antioxidant.

Vitamin E

Like vitamin C, vitamin E is involved in numerous aspects of the body's health. Among its functions, vitamin E assists in the maintenance of a healthy blood vascular system. Vitamin E blocks the oxidation of LDL (the bad cholesterol), preventing it from forming plaque on artery walls, thus reducing the chance of heart attack and stroke, and improving circulation. It also has a strong positive effect on the immune system.

Unlike vitamin C, vitamin E is fat soluble, and is therefore an effective antioxidant among the body's lipids, preventing them from oxidizing and becoming rancid. In addition, vitamin E is most effective in neutralizing polyunsaturated fatty-acid radicals.

In the section on aging we saw that the action of sun on the skin can bring about skin damage. It does this by causing the formation of free radicals, which in turn eat away at the cells and tissues. This damage often manifests itself in the form of wrinkles and age spots.

Because vitamin E is so effective in this area, it is often found as a component in lotions, creams, and other skin care products.

Through its traditionally recognized functions, and most importantly through its action as an antioxidant, vitamin E is invaluable to the body's health, and as an agent in the war on aging.

Synergism

For all of their effectiveness as antioxidants when acting on their own, beta-carotene, vitamin C, and vitamin E confer an even stronger, synergistic effect when used in conjunction with one another.

Grape-seed Extract

Grape-seed extract contains a group of compounds called procyanidolic oligomers (PCO), which are part of a larger group called the bioflavonoids.

Although bioflavonoids may occur elsewhere - in the skins of certain fruits, for instance - it is the bioflavonoids that are found in grape-seed extract that exhibit the most powerful and most effective properties as antioxidants. Some have even estimated the efficacy of grape-seed flavonoids at 40 or 50 times that of vitamin E. As a further benefit in this regard, grape-seed extract also enhances the antioxidant effects of vitamins C and E by 20 to 50 times.

Grape-seed extract has also exhibited strong anti-inflammatory properties, which may possibly produce beneficial effects in the treatment of arthritis. Because it blocks the enzyme responsible for producing histamine, grape-seed extract is an excellent anti-allergy, anti-cold remedy as well.

A few years back, red wine was shown to be beneficial in promoting heart health (when taken regularly in the amounts of a glass or two per day. No more!) It is now thought that this benefit is not only due to the alcohol involved, but to the bioflavonoids from the grapes, themselves. These PCO bioflavonoids work against the oxidation of LDL, thereby reducing its ability to form arterial plaque. They also help maintain and increase the elasticity of arteries.

Further, with improved vascular health conferred by these bioflavonoids, comes improved tissue health. One way in which this improved tissue health manifests itself is in the form of healthy gums and teeth. This improved tissue health also shows up in terms of a strengthened and improved immune system.

As was the case for most vitamins (except for vitamin D, produced by the action of sunlight on the skin; and indirectly in the digestive tract, for vitamin K), the body is unable to manufacture bioflavonoids. Therefore, to obtain the strong antioxidant and anti-inflammatory effects brought about by grape-seed extract, a good supplement is strongly recommended.

Table of Antioxidants

1. Vitamins A, E, and C: Excellent free radical scavengers.
2. Proanthocyanidins: Found in grape-seed and pine bark.
3. Herbs: ginkgo biloba, garlic.
4. Quercetin: from zucchini, squash, green tea, garlic.
5. Lycopene: from tomatoes.
6. Minerals: selenium, germanium.
7. Hormones: melatonin, DHEA.
8. Amino Acids: glutathione, methionine, NAC.

Flavonoid Classes

1. Flavonols: from green tea, grape seed, pine bark
2. Proanthocyanidins: from pine bark, grape seed, huckleberries, ginkgo biloba.
3. Flavones: from Quercetin in green tea, garlic.
4. Biflavones: from ginkgo biloba.
5. Flavonones: from hesperidin in citrus peels.
6. Flavononoles: from milk thistle and pine bark.
7. Anthocyanins: from red grapes, wine, huckleberries.
8. Flavonolignans: from milk thistle, artichokes.
9. Isoflavones: from genistein and diadzein of soy beans.

Minerals: Mining The Mother Lode

We are all aware by now of the body's need for minerals such as calcium and iron. If the importance of these minerals to the health of the body were to be put in mining terms, we might say that they are part of the mother lode. There are, however, other minerals, as well, that play an equally important part in the health of the body, and they too might be considered as part of the mother lode.

The three minerals that we will look at here include selenium, magnesium, and chromium. Given the health benefits these minerals bring to us, they are certainly worth our mining.

Selenium

Because selenium is such a strong antioxidant, it could just as readily have been grouped with them. As an antioxidant, it is most effective in neutralizing polyunsaturated fatty-acid radicals. Working in conjunction with glutathione (itself considered to be one of the master intracellular anti-oxidants), selenium - through a process known as chelation - is able to help cleanse the body of toxic heavy metals such as lead, mercury, and cadmium.

Studies have shown that adequate quantities of selenium in the diet also help to diminish the risk of cancer and heart disease, and to strengthen the immune system. Selenium is necessary for the production of *glutathione peroxidase*.

The amount of selenium in the diet depends to a considerable extent on where we live and what we eat. If there is less selenium in the soil of a particular area, there will be less selenium in the foodstuffs grown there.

The better vitamin pills will have selenium, and other minerals, included in their formulation. These are the ones to choose when selecting a multivitamin.

Magnesium

Probably the role many of us are familiar with concerning magnesium is in its frequent combination with calcium. This combination is often used because magnesium promotes a better absorption of calcium by the body. Also, magnesium helps the body to make more efficient use of calcium, allowing calcium to more readily perform its many tasks.

A study done by Penland and P.E. Johnson, as well as another by A. Nicholas, have shown that magnesium may help reduce symptoms of PMS. It is generally thought that magnesium, taken with calcium by women prior to their menstrual periods, may confer even greater efficacy than when either is taken alone. In addition, studies by P.D. Turlapaty and B.M. Altura, as well as L.T. Iseri et al, show that magnesium is important in maintaining heart health.

On its own, magnesium is also a strong antioxidant. It is able to counter the effects of free radicals, especially as they affect the little energy factories in the cell, the mitochondria. By helping protect the mitochondria from free radical damage, magnesium thereby closes off another avenue that leads to aging.

By helping regulate the operating levels of calcium, magnesium plays an indirect role in keeping the heart beating in a normal rhythm. Magnesium is also necessary for the action it has on a host of enzymes in the body.

Because too much magnesium is not good for us, and may induce nausea and vomiting, we are well advised to monitor our intake of magnesium. On the other hand, because of magnesium's necessity to the body, we are equally well advised to get adequate amounts of it.

Chromium

Chromium is another of the "mother lode" minerals. One of the chief benefits of chromium is that it promotes an efficient use of insulin in sugar metabolism. As a consequence, this brings about an efficient metabolizing of glucose - which, in turn, is instrumental in stabilizing blood sugar levels.

Because insulin also affects T-cells and interferon, when insulin is working at peak efficiency, this helps to maintain the immune system in top fighting form. Indirectly, then, chromium plays an important role, as well, in helping to arm the immune system.

Chromium has also been shown to promote lower levels of triglycerides and LDL cholesterol, which is the bad cholesterol. At the same time it promotes higher levels of HDL, the healthy cholesterol. It is not surprising, then, that optimal levels of chromium are conducive to good heart health.

As a further plus, chromium plays an important part in the body's use of protein, and in the formation of muscle tissue.

Chromium has shown itself to be extremely safe when taken in proper quantities. On the other hand, given the benefits of chromium, it is well worth the care in making sure we get enough of it. Several studies have been done to demonstrate the benefits of chromium and we have seen our own anecdotal evidence with our diabetes Type 2 patients when they are marginally controlled with oral medication.

Sundry Supplements

Coenzyme Q-10

Just when you thought you were safely out of the alphabet soup, you now find yourself confronted with coenzyme Q-10, or CoQ-10.

As its name suggests, CoQ-10 has to do with an enzyme. An enzyme is a substance that serves as a catalyst in promoting a specific biochemical reaction. Enzymes consist of a protein component combined with a mineral or vitamin component. The vitamin component is called the coenzyme.

CoQ-10 is a particular coenzyme that is found throughout the body, and in especially high concentrations in the heart and liver. One of its principal functions is to facilitate the conversion of sugars into a compound called adenosine triphosphate, or ATP. ATP is a key player in a complex series of biochemical reactions, whose end result is to supply the body with energy. Put most simply, CoQ-10 helps the body to burn sugar and obtain energy.

CoQ-10 is essential for good heart health. All cardiologists will agree that CoQ-10 will protect the heart from the toxicity of Adriamycin in children. Studies discussed in "Coenzyme Q-10 : Is it Our New Fountain of Youth?" by William H. Lee, have shown that CoQ-10 has been able to bring about strong improvement in treadmill performance in cardiac patients. In another study, patients with congestive heart failure were treated with CoQ-10: four weeks later 53% of them were showing no symptoms at all.

With its involvement in energy production, and its strong presence in the liver, CoQ-10 also promotes good liver health. This is important because the liver plays such a multi-faceted role in the body's well being. One of the liver's important functions is that it is continuously cleansing poisons and pollutants out of the blood. Also, the liver produces bile, which is very important in the digestion of fats.

Other studies discussed in the above mentioned publication have shown that 50% of obese individuals are deficient in CoQ-10. Almost all vegetarians are deficient in CoQ-10. Since CoQ-10 promotes optimal energy production in cells (a process that uses up sugar), and since it also promotes a healthy liver (optimizing its role in the digestion of fats), we should not be surprised to learn that CoQ-10 has been instrumental in promoting weight loss.

CoQ-10 has also been shown to act as an antioxidant, but the detailed functioning in this regard has not yet been determined. So far, it appears that CoQ-10 is able to inhibit the oxidation of fats by free radicals.

In addition, studies have shown that CoQ-10 helps boost the immune system. One study in particular, done by Emile Bliznakov, demonstrated that CoQ-10 brought about a doubling in the rate of phagocytosis in rats. (Phagocytosis is the process whereby white blood cells engulf and remove foreign matter from the blood.)

Another study done on mice showed that, with CoQ-10 treatments, their rate of antibody production was doubled. This brought their antibody production almost in line with that found in young mice.

Since the levels of CoQ-10 in the body tend to diminish with age, for those approaching their 50's, this is a supplement worth looking into. However, CoQ-10 has produced some instances of diarrhea and nausea, suggesting that it should be taken in appropriate dosages, and under the care and monitoring of a medical doctor. Patients taking statin drugs for cholestorol problems have decreased CoQ-10, levels possibly adding to their fatigue.

Ginkgo Biloba

Ginkgo biloba refers to an extract made from the leaves of the Gingko biloba tree. Because it has shown excellent results in improving circulation, particularly in the brain, it has often been used as a memory booster.

Research based in Germany has shown that geriatric patients treated with gingko biloba extract achieved improved results on psychometric tests. These same patients receiving gingko biloba extract also exhibited an improved and more positive frame of mind. In our practice, Ginkgo has helped with vertigo (dizziness) perhaps by improving blood flow to the labyrinth apparatus of the ear.

Other research done in England showed that gingko biloba treatments brought about an improvement in adults with mild to moderate memory loss.

The accumulated results of studies like these suggest that gingko may have the capability of delaying the onset, or diminishing the memory loss, that invariably accompanies Alzheimer's disease.

In publications by E. Murray ("Gingko Biloba: the Amazing 200 Million Year Old Healer") and D.B. Mowrey ("Herbal Tonic Therapies"), further benefits of gingko biloba are set forth. Gingko biloba extract has shown that in its capacity to ease bronchial constriction, it can limit and ameliorate asthma attacks. Also, and probably related to gingko biloba's ability to improve blood flow, gingko has been shown to improve male sexual function.

Since a number of the conditions that gingko biloba has been effective in treating are also those associated with the aging process, gingko biloba may be the perfect supplement for those getting along in years. You must check with your doctor before taking Ginko Biloba. It may interfere with blood clotting.

Echinacea

At one time it seems that no one in North America had ever heard of Echinacea - now it appears that everyone has. Most preparations of Echinacea are derived from a plant called *Echinacea angustifolia*, although sometimes other varieties may be used. Many gardeners may know the plant as the purple coneflower. North American Indians called it the snake plant, and used it to counteract poisons from snake and insect bites. It is generally the root from the plant that is used, either dried, or as an extract or juice. Oddly, although the plant is native to North America, much of the initial research done on it has been done in Germany.

Echinacea is well known for an ability to fortify the body against colds and flu. It may be a strong booster to the body's immune system and, as well, it may be an effective anti-inflammatory.   As an anti-inflammatory it has been used for years in alleviating the suffering of arthritis.

Imedeen

Imedeen is a new oral antioxidant treatment for photo aged skin as researched by Charles Lynde of the University of Toronto. It is a combination of antioxidants and is an example of future super-antioxidant products, one of which Dr.'s White and McLeod are currently developing to increase superoxide dismutase (S.O.D.) and catalase, perhaps the most important antioxidants in the cells.

Dr. Ranjeet Chandra of Memorial University Canada, found that patients taking supplements of vitamins and trace minerals had significant improvement in recent memory, abstractability, problem solving and attention span.

We have also studied our patients to find positive effects of combining antioxidant vitamins with statin drugs for those treated for cholesterol problems.

More information about antioxidants and their future promise will be found in our new book available in 2002, titled, *Doctors' Secrets – The Antioxidant Highway.*

Immunocal

Immunocal is an un-denatured whey protein developed at McGill University in Montreal, and is showing promise as a supplement to elevate intracellular glutathione levels.

SECTION VI

Conclusion

*"If a man takes no thought about what is distant,
he will find sorrow near at hand."*

– Confucius *(lived 80 years)*

*"And the Lord said, 'My Spirit shall not always strive
with man, or that he also is flesh: yet his days
shall be one hundred and twenty years.'*

– Genesis: Chapter 6, Verse 3

*"Sloppy, raggedy-assed old life. I love it.
I never want to die."*

– Dennis Trudell

*"I don't want to achieve immortality through my work,
I want to achieve it through not dying."*

– Woody Allen

*"I am not afraid to die.
I just don't want to be there when it happens."*

– Woody Allen

*"The one advantage of living to 120 years:
No peer pressure."*

Conclusion

PRESCRIPTIONS FOR WELLNESS AND LONGEVITY

Not Enough Jets

An acquaintance once told us about a man who, each morning, used to come down to the hot tub in their apartment complex. The man was somewhere in his late 50's and in obviously failing health.

He would hobble over to the hot tub, slowly make his way down the steps, and painfully settle himself into the hot water. Then, for the next half hour, he would strain this way and that, trying to get various parts of his body in front of first one, and then another, of the jets. And every morning he would utter the same lament: "Not enough jets. There's just not enough jets."

We do not want to reach the ripe old age of a hundred plus years if the last third of them are going to be in this kind of debilitating ill health. If we are going to extend our life span, we want that extended time to be filled with vigor and mobility. We want that time to be filled with meaningful activity. We want that time to be filled with wellness.

The authors wish there was a word that embodied the idea of going into an extended life span in wonderfully good health - perhaps something like "wellgevity". Such a word would also have connotations of happy fulfillment.

And that is what we wish to address here - our thoughts on a mode of living that will promote such a possibility, that will grant us those extra years and decades in a body that is replete with wellness. Because if we can gain those extra years and decades, we want them filled with energy and satisfaction. We want them filled with joyous pursuits and fulfillment. We do not want them filled with a glassy eyed stare out a window onto nothingness We do not want them filled with hobbling and pain. Most of all, we do not want them filled with mornings like those of the old man in the hot tub - starting each day with the lament: "Not enough jets!"

Two Fast Tracks to the Grave

If we look over the earlier material in this book we will see that there are two broad avenues of aging, both speeding us along to our final destination in the earth. We might regard them as the two fast tracks to the grave.

The first fast track has to do with the general decline in hormone levels as we approach middle age. The second fast track involves the accumulated damage inflicted on cells and tissues over the years by free radicals.

Of course, there are other factors involved as well, factors over which we have no control. We do not, at the present time, have an effective way of curtailing the shortening of the telomeres that takes place when our cells undergo cell division. (And more on that shortly.) There is also the matter of our individual genetic inheritance: we have no control over a genetic predisposition to accumulating fat rather than remaining slim, or being at higher risk for this or that disease; but in the future we might well be able to modify it. More on this shortly as well.

But two major factors taking us to age and decrepitude - hormone depletion and free radical damage - we can change. We can change and we must change - if we wish to get off the fast track to the grave.

But the time to embark on a wellness and longevity program is not when we are approaching the deathbed. It is too late then. The time to embark on a program of wellness is now, while we are still in reasonably good health. Because then it is simply a matter of regaining a bit of lost ground, and thereafter maintaining these gains, of maintaining our good health, and enjoying the extra couple decades we can gain by turning back the clock.

The Magnificent Seven Prescriptions for Longevity

Prescription # 1:

Hormone Replacement, Particularly HGH

We have seen that hormone replacement is an extremely effective way of countering so many aspects of aging. When we bring the hormones back to youthful levels, we bring much of our body chemistry back as well. Such a program, if begun before too much of the aging process has taken place, may not keep us alive forever. But the evidence does indicate that it may well extend our lives by another couple of decades. And it will give us those decades in relatively good health, in a body that will remain youthful and energetic.

All hormone replacement should be done under the care and monitoring of a medical doctor. This is especially so if there is a particular hormone deficiency such as thyroid hormone deficiency. Age reversal doctors or anti-aging physicians have a particular interest in the field which deals with maintaining correct hormonal balances. However, these services are not generally covered by many medical plans.

We have seen that one of the best ways of keeping the hormonal levels in the youthful range, and of keeping our cellular physiology in the youthful range, is by keeping our levels of HGH in a youthful range. One of the simplest ways of doing that is by the use of secretogogues, which doesn't require a doctor. We will recall that we can stimulate the pituitary to release more HGH and bring the levels back to those of bygone years by use of secretogogues. This does not require great

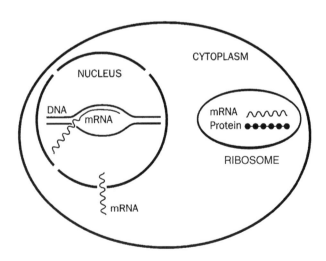

*mRNA (messenger RNA) leaves the nucleus
from the DNA to make proteins in the ribosomes.
HGH stimulates this process through IGF-1.*

expense, nor trips to a clinic for repeated injections. And because these secretogogues are simply stimulating the pituitary to do what it normally does, the HGH levels are then controlled by the body's feedback loop, and will not exceed normal levels. This makes secretogogue use an extremely safe therapy as well.

In our opinion, the use of secretogogues is one of the simplest, safest, least expensive, and most convenient ways of raising and maintaining the levels of HGH in the body to which the majority will respond. Which makes it the easiest way of maintaining a youthful physiology.

So prescription # 1 is: Maintain youthful levels of hormones in the body, and most particularly, maintain youthful levels of HGH.

Prescription # 2:

Maintain High Levels of Antioxidants

We have seen that the cumulative damage done by free radicals is a major factor in bringing about our physical deterioration, and eventual death. We have also seen that the best way of preventing this damage is by making sure we get sufficient antioxidants to neutralize these rampaging free radicals within us.

The diets of most people today are generally inadequate. They are inadequate not only in what they supply - or don't supply - by way of antioxidants, but in other respects as well. Because so much of our food is over-processed it has been depleted of much of its nutritional value. And because of the hectic pace of modern living, we often do not eat wisely or well.

(Further exacerbating the problem, our modern environment - by way of pollution, increased UV rays, etc. - invariably brings about increased free radical activity in our bodies.)

One of the simplest ways of making up much of the nutritional shortfall is through the use of appropriate supplements, and most particularly, of those supplements which raise the levels of antioxidants in our bodies. Here again, there is a simple and inexpensive way of achieving this: by taking a superior quality multivitamin every day. Since vitamins cost only a dollar or so per day, it is worth paying a bit more to get the best vitamin formulation you can. In addition to the vitamins, these formulations will also contain the major minerals the body needs, including the "mother lode" minerals that also serve as powerful antioxidants. To increase your intake of antioxidants to even higher levels, you might want further supplements of beta-carotene or grape-seed extract or a catalase or a superoxide dismutase. Newer products like Microhydrin (silica cage antioxidant) developed by Dr. Flanagan have shown promise.

So, to slow the aging process that comes from free radical damage to the cells of the body, prescription #2 is: Maintain strong levels of antioxidants in the body.

Prescription # 3:

Eat Sensibly

If you are raising your levels of HGH to youthful levels, and are taking adequate quantities of antioxidants, then it would make sense to embrace a sensible diet as well. HGH will promote the building up of muscle and the loss of fat no matter what, but it will do a far better job if a reasonable diet is added to the mix

The same can be said with respect to the anti-oxidants. If we want them to do their job most effectively, we would be well advised to stay away from junk food loaded with preservatives and chemicals, as well as foods that are obvious carcinogens (cancer producers), such as meats loaded with nitrites. As a corollary, we would do well to include foods rich in antioxidants in our diets.

A strong priority in setting up a sensible diet is to keep the total number of calories we take in limited to what we need. All calories are derived from proteins, carbohydrates and fats. We have seen that on a diet where calories are extremely restricted, the aging process is slowed. For those not inclined to that degree of abstemiousness, a more moderate, and more achievable goal, is to keep our caloric needs met, and no more.

Another reason for managing the calories wisely is that, although HGH tends to promote fat loss regardless, the levels of HGH tend to be lower in people who are obese. So it makes sense to try and assist HGH in its work by restricting the caloric intake to a reasonable level, and to try and maintain a physique that is fairly devoid of extra fat. This will not only assist HGH in keeping the body lean and muscled, it will greatly benefit our cardiovascular health, and our overall health in virtually every other respect.

Since HGH promotes the production of muscle mass, it is imperative that we provide the building blocks the body will need to do this. These building blocks come from the protein we digest and break down into

amino acids. There are many sources of protein, but two
of the better ones are chicken and fish. In the case of
some fish, such as salmon or mackerel, the omega 3 oils
will also assist in combating the bad cholesterol.

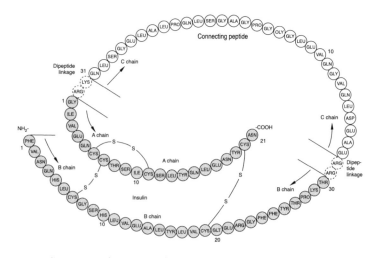

*Structure of PRO Insulin (Human) with A and B chains
that will combine to form insulin*

It is unlikely that North Americans ever get too
little by way of carbohydrates in the diet. However, a
sensible diet will include complex carbohydrates such as
are found in fruits, vegetables, and whole grains, and will
exclude refined carbohydrates such as candy, sugar, and
so on. The glycemic index of carbohydrates is a
reflection of how quickly carbs can induce insulin
secretion from the pancreas. The low index carbs are
preferable to keep the insulin levels low normal by
keeping blood sugar low also. High insulin levels will
effect other hormones and can lead onto insulin
resistance, obesity and Diabetes Type 2. Biguanide drugs
like Metformin and newer thiazolidinediones like
Roziglitazone and Pioglitazone may be of great benefit in
preventing wild swings in blood sugar and insulin levels

in the aging impaired glucose intolerant patients.

Probably the most important thing the average North American can do to improve his or her diet is to get more of fruits and vegetables, and in as wide a variety as possible. This will immediately put more vitamins, minerals, antioxidants, and anti-carcinogens into the body. Most fruits and vegetables also contain considerable quantities of fibre, which is important in keeping the muscles in the intestines toned and working well. In addition, quantities of fibre take longer for the digestive tract to process and therefore keep us feeling full for longer periods of time.

Another important thing the average North American can do to immediately improve his or her diet is to cut down on fats. There are fats and saturated oils hidden in many products on the shelves these days, so ferreting them out may take some vigilance. Turning to chicken, turkey or toxin free fish will help cut down on the fat intake. Substituting with fruits and vegetables will do even more. Diets high in free fatty acids (too much omega-6 like sunflower and safflower oil) combined with high levels of insulin will increase levels of arachidonic acid and raise levels of bad eicosanoids (short range hormones) which will mediate inflammation and pain at the cellular level. "On the other hand," (Randy Travis, Merritt 2000) raising omega-3 fatty acids (fish oils) raise the good eicosapentanoic acid levels to balance the bad eicosanoids. In summary, eat hormonally neutral mono-unsaturated fats (olives, nuts) so that cell membrane permeability is not affected for nutrients, antioxidants and hormones.

Water is something we rarely think about as being part of our diet, but it is a very necessary part. It is especially so since many of the liquids that we drink each day are diuretics, which means that they tend to increase the flow of urine. Things like coffee, tea, and alcohol are all diuretics. When you consume these beverages you may actually end up with a net loss of water in the body. This makes it all the more important that you drink plenty of water each day. Taking in enough water will ensure that dehydration does not become a problem, and it will provide an ideal internal medium in which the body can effect its countless chemical reactions. It will also allow you to better flush out toxins during exercise. At least 8 glasses of pure water (sometimes alkalinized) each day is recommended.

To amplify or assist your efforts in providing the body with optimal nutrient intake, you may want to consider supplements of one kind or another. This is especially so where you feel that your diet is inadequate for any reason: hectic schedule; poor eating habits that are hard to break; insufficient variety in the diet. You may also want to consider supplements if you have special dietary needs, such as may occur for those involved in weight training, body building, or any other form of heavy exercise. If you are on a strict diet for the purposes of losing weight, you will almost certainly want to think about supplements.

Because so much of the North American diet consists of processed foods, so much of it provides limited nutrition. This situation makes supplements almost a necessity for some people, if they are to get all the nutrients they need. For others, given the hectic pace of daily life - and its tendency to induce poor eating habits - many will at least want to consider a good multivitamin. This will be one that also includes the mother lode minerals. Depending on circumstance, others, still, will perhaps need additional antioxidants as well.

In summing up, then, take in only the number of calories you need to maintain your desired weight. Strive for a balanced diet that includes a wide variety of foodstuffs - meats, whole grains products, and dairy. Most importantly, make sure you get plenty of fruits and vegetables. Just as important, if you are on HGH replacement therapy, by capsule secretagogues, or HGH injections, make certain you get sufficient protein for the body to use in building up that increased muscle mass.

To put it all even more succinctly, as prescription #3: Eat sensibly.

In fact much of today's dietary literature promotes protein loading at supper with an evening fast, to encourage HGH release.

Prescription # 4:

Get Enough Exercise

The body is like a machine in that it has to be run, or it runs down. It has to be active or it will atrophy.

Most of us have seen what happens when a broken arm or a leg is immobilized in a cast. After the cast is removed some weeks or months later, invariably the limb is visibly smaller and weaker than its counterpart. Another example of USE IT OR LOSE IT.

There are numerous benefits to be obtained from exercise. For one thing, exercise builds muscle. Also, we have seen that exercise - especially strenuous exercise - increases the levels of HGH in the body. This makes strenuous exercise an excellent adjunct to HGH replacement therapy, especially when secretogogues are employed.

Exercise and fidgeting also burns off fat, which sets up a cyclical effect we looked at earlier: HGH helps us to shed fat, and when we shed fat our levels of HGH tend to be higher, which then helps us shed even more fat. And so on.

When we exercise and burn off fat (converted into sugar), we set in motion a biochemical process that, in a sense, runs in the opposite direction of the biochemistry that turns sugar into fat. You might think of the process as something of a conveyor belt which, when it is running one way, peels off fat molecules and converts them into sugar, which are then to be burnt off to produce energy. Going in the opposite direction, the conveyor belt takes sugar molecules, turns them into fat, and stores them. If through exercise, you get the conveyor belt going rapidly in the direction that is burning off fat, it keeps going that way for some time even after you have stopped exercising. It is as if the body builds up a metabolic momentum that keeps the process going for some time afterwards on its own. Which explains why people who exercise can generally eat more in calories than they burn off with the exercise, and still remain slim. They have pushed their bodies into a more efficient sugar metabolism, which continues to work in that mode even when they are not exercising.

Obviously, then, exercise is a natural accompaniment to dieting. If, through exercise, you can press the body into a more efficient sugar metabolism, you will not have to watch over every last calorie. This means that every so often you can have your extra piece of cake and eat it too. And you can overindulge now and again in other ways without fretting, because the exercise will take care of those occasional extra calories. So if you are at a party some evening and have more to eat and drink than your diet allows, not to worry. Your pumped up muscles and your pumped up metabolism will be putting them on the conveyor belt to the furnace. We have all noticed this in our friends that are in great shape.

Exercise also tends to flush the system of toxins, especially the heavy metals. Here, again, we see why adequate water intake is so important.

Where hard, strenuous exercise will raise HGH levels in the body, aerobic exercise is of great benefit to the heart and lungs. However, both kinds of exercise bring about the formation of more free radicals in the body, which means that when you are on an exercise program you should increase still further your intake of antioxidants.

Because exercise helps keep us healthy, and helps us to live longer and live stronger, prescription #4 is: Get enough exercise.

Prescription # 5 :

Take Care of Your Immune System

You must maintain an excellent body hygiene. Any chronic infections must be eliminated by any means. Bad teeth, parasites in the bowel, bacterial and viral infections must all be treated with either herbal or conventional means with your doctor.

Prescription # 6:

Reduce Stress, Enhance Spirituality

Many stressors stimulate the release of ACTH (adrenocorticotropin hormone, 39 amino acids) from the anterior pituitary gland, via stimulation from the hypothalamus peptide, corticotropin releasing hormone (CRH). ACTH increases HGH output but also increases cortisone output from the adrenal gland which ultimately suppresses DHEA production.

Fulfillment of Spiritualism is a necessity for relaxation and satisfaction of the mind. The mind - body connection is not complete unless the spirit is satisfied.

Prescription # 7:

Detoxification

Detoxification of the poisons bathing our bodies from our environment is a necessity. Through the cytochrome P450 system and hydroxylation and conjugation reactions in the liver, gut and kidney we are better able to handle the toxins. We encourage only modest alcohol consumption and promote clean, washed food and amino acid supplements.

These prescriptions, although simple and relatively easy to follow, can add years - decades, even - to your life. More importantly, they increase immensely the prospect of having those extra years and decades filled with wellness and activity.

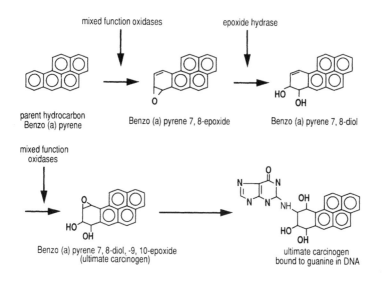

Some Cancer causing agents Benzo (A) Pyrene which binds to DNA

Overview and Summation

We have seen that our hormone levels tend to decline sharply from about the time of middle age onwards, and that this decline in hormone levels plays a key role in bringing on the aging process. From the work of Dr. Chein and Dr. Terry at the Palm Springs Life Extension Institute we have also seen that by employing hormone replacement therapy - and most particularly by the use of HGH replacement therapy - that many aspects of aging can be halted, or even reversed. HGH, when returned to youthful levels in the body, is able to bring back a youthful physiology - it is able to turn back the clock. This reversal of the aging process manifests itself outwardly in numerous ways: fat loss, muscle gain, improved sexual performance and pleasure, the reduction or elimination of wrinkles, and on and on.

These kinds of results were also obtained in studies done by Dr. Bengtsson in Sweden, and by other researchers in Europe and America. In Dr. Rudman's initial study, where HGH was administered to men in their 60's and 70's, the results were truly amazing. With the obvious improvements that the HGH treatment brought about - fat loss, muscle gain, rejuvenation of skin and hair - some of the patients appeared to have had their aging process rolled back 10 or 20 years. For them, HGH had turned back the clock a decade or two. And these were men in their 60's and 70's, men who were already well along the downward spiral of aging.

For men and women heading into their forties and fifties, the authors cannot help but feel that the results will be even more amazing yet. In most of these people, the aging process is just beginning to make itself felt, the decay has not gone that far yet. Here, HGH can counter the aging process early in its evolution, before the decay has become fully entrenched. You might liken it to getting to a dentist before the cavity in the tooth has decayed too much of it. When the cavity is caught and filled early on, the tooth will be strong and will last a long time. But when the tooth is drilled and filled only after the cavity has rotted half the tooth, that tooth will probably not last nearly so long.

So, for people in their 40's and 50's, even many in their 60's, the evidence so far suggests to us that HGH replacement can add a decade or two - perhaps even more - to the expected life span. And we are not talking about merely being alive, merely existing, trying to find a hot tub with still more jets. We are talking about these extra years, these extra decades being filled with wellness, with energy, with activity.

And when you add antioxidants to the picture, the prospects become even brighter. And when you then add a pattern of sensible eating habits, and throw in a 30 minute session of exercise done about 3 times a week, then we think that adding an extra 30 years of reasonably healthy living to the expected life span is perhaps even something of a conservative estimate.

A Simple, Easy Program

The program we are proposing here is not a difficult, costly, or prohibitive program. In fact, it is quite simple, and within the reach and capability of most people in North America today. It begins with returning HGH levels to youthful levels. If this is done by using secretogogues, it means there will be no injections necessary, and no ongoing trips to a clinic. You simply take a few capsules just before bedtime that will stimulate the pituitary to release increased amounts of HGH after you fall asleep.

The second part - maintaining optimal levels of antioxidants in the body - is equally simple. Most of the antioxidants may be obtained from a top quality multi-vitamin pill. To this, further supplements such as catalase and superoxide dismutase will soon be available.

The third part involves keeping to a clean sensible diet that includes sufficient protein, as well as a proper variety of fruits and vegetables. Add to this a pattern of not overeating, and you are near the end of the list. Reduction of stress by relaxation techniques, proper hygiene, detoxification when necessary, getting in touch with your spiritual self and you are almost done.

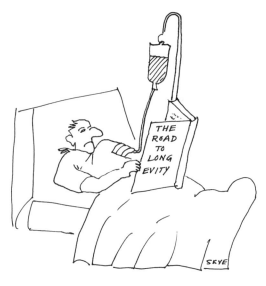

"The Procrastinator"

All that is left now, is a bit of exercise. Strengthening workouts in 30 minute sessions, done approximately every second day and now the program is complete.

Make it Fun

Maintaining optimal levels of HGH and antioxidants in the body is merely a matter of taking a few pills a day. As for diet and exercise, this can be easy too - if you make it fun. After all, not only do we want to add these extra years and decades to our lives, and not only do we want them to filled with wellness, we also want them to be filled with meaning and happiness.

Eating, for instance, should never be dreary or dull. In the past twenty years, accompanying the increased interest in health, there have been hundreds of cookbooks published, many of which aim at providing not only healthy meals, but meals that tickle the taste buds. There is everything from the hearty to the exotic, from Italian to Thai. So there is no need for meals to be difficult or dull.

And since you can have meals that are both good tasting and good for you, why not? The two are no longer mutually exclusive.

As for overeating, if that has been your pattern, try to include more vegetables and fruits in your meals. They will help fill you up without inflicting nearly as many calories as you will get from most meals. More than anything, try leaving the table after your first helping. Try going for a walk instead of going for a second helping. Take a short stroll to a nearby park or plaza, instead of lolling about on the couch, feeling like a python that has swallowed a pig. You will actually feel lighter and more energized. And more alive.

Exercise, too, will add to your feeling of being alive. Again, the main thing is to make it enjoyable, not a task. If you are in reasonably good shape, you might want to include some vigorous exercise. For example, if you are playing tennis, try putting a dollar on the match. It will certainly increase your enjoyment and interest in the match, and your energy output. If you do some jogging, try to finish with a strong kick. This will bump the aerobic aspect up a notch, and help increase HGH levels. Ditto for swimming. After those leisurely lengths at the pool, finish up with a few speed lengths that leave you panting. If you want to really work on those muscles, try to add some weight training to your program. Be careful of injuries associated with extreme sports or body contact exercises, but we love our hockey and squash!

The most important thing, however, is to choose the kinds of exercise that you can enjoy. If you enjoy it, you will stick with it. One of the best ways to make any activity more enjoyable is to do it with someone. So if you go for a jog, do it with a spouse, a soul-mate, a friend. If you tend to get bored with one kind of exercise, do more than one kind. Vary your routine. You are in it for the long haul, so, whatever you do, make it fun. That way, you will stick with it.

The Payoff

What we have described above is not a hard program. You take a few capsules (secretogogues) before bed; you take a multivitamin that includes minerals with one of your meals (and additional supplements where required); you engage in exercise that you enjoy about three times a week; and without overeating, you eat and enjoy tasty, yet nutritious meals, with a glass or two of red wine thrown in for good measure.

This is hardly a tough regimen. In fact, 80 % of the world's population would love the chance to embrace such a program just for the food alone, because it would mean they would finally get enough to eat. And for many, it would mean less exercise, not more. And it would mean a pleasurable kind of exercise, not pick and shovel exercise.

Also, this is a flexible and forgiving program. If you overeat here and there, the exercise will probably take care of those extra calories. If you miss the occasional exercise session, the sensible eating will maintain the physique. And the optimal HGH and antioxidant levels will continue with the physiological maintenance when diet or exercise are interrupted, as may happen during a vacation or illness. So if any aspect of the program becomes interrupted briefly, it's not like falling off the wagon. You simply resume it from where you left off. Because you are in it for the long haul.

And that's the payoff: you are in it for the long haul: you gain an extra twenty or thirty years - years of wellness and good health.

The average life expectancy for Americans is approaching 80 years of age, and this includes those who smoke, do drugs; who go for the fattiest of pork chops and eat two or three of them at a sitting; who are extremely sedentary, drink large quantities of alcohol, coffee, and soft drinks, and in general just don't take care of themselves. If people with these lifestyles are included in the total population, and this total population still has an average life expectancy of about 76 years or better, then we do not think it unreasonable to conclude that, on average, those following a program such as we have described above, will make it to 100 or 120 years of age, and exercising under their own steam.

What Those Extra Years Really Mean

To say you will have an extra twenty or thirty years of wellness and activity does not give much of a picture of what this really means. Taken on their own like that, they are just numbers. But what they really mean is that you will finally have the time to do so many of the things that you could never fit in to your busy schedule. And you will still be in good shape, and able to undertake these activities fully.

For example, if the demands of career and family have kept you from ever taking a sea cruise, now you will be able to. And you will not be confined to the lounge or a deck chair, but will be frolicking in the pool, or dancing the night away.

Travel of all kinds will be open to you. And because

of your superior good health you will possibly be able to outlast the tour guide through the activities and walkabouts during the day, and still have energy left for a full evening afterwards.

Or perhaps you have always wanted to start up a business, perhaps a little cottage industry, or something on the Internet, but never had the time. Well, now you'll have two or three decades. (We know CEO's in America running companies, to the family's dismay, at age 100 years.)

Or perhaps you've put off writing that book you always felt you had in you. You will then have time to write volumes.

The range of things you can do with those extra years is bound only by your desires. It will be your happy choice to make.

Of course, there will be a statistical few that may not get the full allotment of these extra years. Perhaps a genetic predisposition to this or that disease will make itself felt in spite of the program. If so, you will in any case have made it much farther than you would have otherwise. And there is the possibility that, having made it that much farther along, the genetic predisposition may at that point in time be amenable to correction. But we are getting ahead of ourselves here - more on that point shortly.

Most of you, at any rate, will get those extra decades, and they will be yours in a well functioning body. What you do with them will be limited only by your dreams.

A Deeper Meaning

Although you will want to engage in many activities that you have enjoyed all your life, and especially those that you had to limit or put off altogether, our guess is that in time, for most of you, they will eventually come to be of secondary importance. For those of you who have offspring, they, and their children - your grandchildren - will come to be a primary focus of your extended time.

Certainly, you will continue with your various activities of interest. But a great deal of your time will more than likely come to be spent in family pursuits. We say this because we have seen this pattern occur in patients and in others around us over the years. People hit their 50's, 60's, and 70's and suddenly family ties - even where they had formerly been loose and sporadic - come to the fore. This is especially so when grandchildren arrive.

Just as you did not know beforehand how having a child could transform your life, and bring a new kind of love with its own limitless dimension, you also cannot know how being a grandparent will have its own captivating effect on you. And the attachment and love you will come to feel for your grandchildren will be much like the love you felt for your own children when they came into your life.

Only here, unlike many grandparents in the past, you will not be tucked away in your easy chair in the living room, or in the rocking chair out on the porch - although such happy moments will also be there from time to time. But you will also be able to take those beautiful little creatures and do a host of things with them: teach them to swim, or ride a bike, or play tennis.

Unlike most grandparents of the past, your activities will be almost unlimited. Further, you will be there for your grandchildren not only through childhood, but you will be there for them through their teenage years, well able to serve as guide and mentor during this difficult and formative period.

Then, in twenty year's time, when they in turn have children, you will still be in sufficient good health and good shape, to do it all again with the great-grandchildren. You will still be sufficiently mobile to do a great many things with them, again teaching them and guiding them in a difficult and complicated world. And where the parents may at times be too rushed or stressed, with your time, patience, and experience you may be better situated to help these future generations than anyone else. In fact, helping them to unfurl their sails and gently puff them with wind, and helping them set the rudder so as to steer through the shoals, may turn out to be some of the more rewarding experiences of your life.

And when their children arrive, and you are perhaps a hundred or a hundred plus years of age, you will be there to welcome them, too - your great-great-grandchildren - into the world. By this time the more vigorous activities may be denied you, but you will - most of you - still be able to do a great many things with this generation as well.

Enjoying these future generations, serving as mentor and guide, may well come to be the focal point of your life. But you will, of course, keep up with other activities you enjoy as well - tennis, swimming, hiking, travel, golf, and so on. All of this goes without saying. But there is another dimension to these years that may also come to play a significant part in your extended time on earth - at least for many of you. And it involves changes we have observed in a great many people as they come upon a certain age.

A Higher Meaning

It has been said that youth is wasted on the young. We do not think that "wasted" is quite the right word. We think, perhaps, that youth is not fully appreciated by the young. By its very nature, youth has little experience and little background upon which to draw in dealing with the world. The advancing years, in contrast, often hold a wide range of experience, experience that confers a certain patience, a serenity, a wisdom.

This serenity, this wisdom, has been described by many to have its underpinning in the feeling that all things are somehow inter-connected, that they all make up one vast, magnificent whole. And accompanying this feeling, very often, is a desire to give something back, to take some of the good that has accrued and give it back to the world. This may show up in a variety of ways: the setting up of scholarships; the volunteering of one's experience and expertise to charitable organizations, and helping in the political arena with invaluable wisdom.

Now, if you are forty or forty something, most of you will probably not have given much thought to this phase of existence. You are busy with family life and with careers that are approaching their zenith. But, as has happened with many in the past, that later stage of life will likely bring a similar outlook to many of you as well. You too, will at some point want to give something back to in some way improve the world around you. If so, you will have a strong advantage. Where those in the past usually had only a few years to improve the lot of their families and their communities, years that were often marred with the increasing ravages of age, you will have many years, decades even, in which to pursue goals that let you give something back.

In essence, then, what those extra years and decades mean is that you will be able to pursue a multitude of activities you hadn't sufficient time for in the past. You will be able to launch projects and dreams that have long been dormant. You will be able to serve as mentor and guide to grandchildren and great-grandchildren. You will have those extra years in which to give back to the world, if you so desire, some of the good you have received from it.

Most importantly, you will have that extra time that will take you to future developments in the field of anti-aging. The importance of the last point is this: we are witnessing a time in which there has been a virtual avalanche of activity in anti-aging research. What was a mere trickle in the 80's and early 90's is now a thundering rush. The information is pouring in, from fields as diverse as nutrition, gerontology, oncology, genetics. Few are the discoveries made these days that do not have application somehow to the field of anti-aging. Most of us do not have the time or patience to wait for more clinical trials and studies.

With this pell-mell surge of furious activity and research, our knowledge about the body, and about the aging process, is growing at an exponential rate. Almost certainly this means that in the next ten and twenty years there will be numerous breakthroughs, some of them stunning, momentous breakthroughs.

By adding these extra years and decades to your life, and by keeping in good shape, not only will you have the enjoyment of those years, you will be there to benefit from the breakthroughs in research that will be coming at you in the future.

The Future

The future is unfolding at breakneck speed. Maybe it's just that there seems to be more of it. Especially in the field of anti-aging. Few discoveries are made these days that do not have some impact on the human life span. Everything from red wine to telomeres to the mapping of the human genome - all tie in one way or another with human longevity.

Each time some discovery is made, it offers yet another way of extending the life span by a little bit. And then every once in a while something big like HGH breaks onto the scene and offers the possibility of extending our lives by a quantum leap.

It is discoveries of this sort that have ignited research in the field of anti-aging and set it expanding like a prairie fire. Adding fuel to this fire is the constant possibility of cross fertilization, where a discovery in one branch of science sets off new pathways of research in others. So when a discovery is made that deals with hormones, it may suggest something to be researched in genetics, or nutrition. Similarly for all other fields - each new discovery leads to a host of others.

What this means is that with the coming advances over the next ten, twenty, or thirty years, if you have kept yourself alive and in good shape you will be able to avail yourself of the benefits these new discoveries bring, which will likely extend your life that much further again. And then you will be there to avail yourself of still further discoveries made in that more distant period of time. And on and on.

Although major discoveries will be made in many fields over the next few years and the next few decades, the areas that currently show immense promise are some of those that we have already touched on in this book. However, it will probably be of interest to take a further tantalizing glimpse of what some of these future discoveries will entail. Because, if you are not interested in longevity now, at age forty, by age sixty you surely will be, most of you, anyway.

Hormones

One of the fields where significant breakthroughs are expected is one where important breakthroughs have already taken place - in the field of hormones.

We have seen, for example, that much work on HGH is still being done, with more data accumulating all the time. For example, it is now known that hormones, including HGH, may regulate the telomerase gene to produce telomerase.

Some of the current research involves raising HGH levels by use of growth hormone releasing hormone (GHRH). Other research has to do with Insulin-like growth factor 1 (IGF-1), the physiological successor of HGH. It is in the form of IGF-1, we will recall, that HGH does much of its work at the various receptor sites in the body.

But IGF-1 is only one of many growth factors being investigated. Other growth factors being looked at today, some of which consist of strings of peptides, produce a wide variety of effects throughout the body. As more work is done with them, we may see them being used in such wide ranging applications as rejuvenating cells damaged by trauma, or in treating burns and ulcers, or in regenerating nerve cells.

Research is also going on in the area of secretogogues, the thrust being to come up with an even more efficient one for the future, but this may prove difficult. One group of substances that shows some promise in this regard consists of growth hormone releasing peptides. Two of these, GHRP 6 and its successor GHRP 2, have shown that they are very effective at stimulating raised levels of growth hormone. Another substance, called hexarelin, has shown a similar effectiveness at raising HGH levels. All are being researched intensively at this time but will be available surely as pharmaceuticals in several years, requiring prescriptions.

Another intriguing idea that has surfaced in regard to hormone research involves a hypothetical hormone that has yet to be discovered. The evidence for this undiscovered hormone is indirect, and puts one in mind of the indirect evidence that led to the discovery of the planet Neptune in 1846. In the latter case, observations had shown that there were perturbations (irregularities) in the orbit of Uranus (the favourite planet of our teenagers) A French mathematician and astronomer named Leverrier concluded that these perturbations were due to the gravitational effects of another - as yet undiscovered - planet that was out beyond Uranus. Leverrier calculated where this undiscovered planet should be to produce the observed gravitational effects on Uranus, and when it was searched for, the planet that came to be known as Neptune was found in the predicted location.

In a similar way, indirect evidence suggests that there is an as yet undiscovered hormone that may effect the decline in HGH levels as we age. Research so far shows that this decline is not solely due to the effects of growth hormone releasing hormone (GHRH) and somatostatin. So quite possibly, some of this decline is due to the action of some unknown hormone. Supporting this idea is the following train of thought. GHRH, produced by the body, works on a particular receptor site in effecting the release of HGH. Man made substances, however, such as GHRP 6, GHRP 2, and hexarelin, which stimulate HGH release as well, effect this release by working at a different receptor site. But there is no known hormone made by the body that works at this second receptor site. The conclusion is obvious. If there is a receptor site, then it must be there for a reason: there must be a hormone produced in the body that does its work there - only it hasn't been discovered yet. This is analogous to a receptor being present for Valium which initially had no known human made substance to fill this receptor. If that turns out to be the case, then perhaps this hormone can be manipulated to keep HGH levels in the optimal range as we age, preventing the decline they normally show in our thirties and forties. Were that to come about we would have yet another arrow in the quiver.

Another question that future research will likely focus on: Is there an HGH resistance that affects us with age analogous to a type of insulin resistance? Maybe as we keep the IGF-1 levels elevated, we may experience some of this as a Somapause Type 2, different from a primary or HGH deficient Somapause Type 1 that we all face with aging.

What we have seen here is but a sampling of the wide ranging research going on in the field of hormones. Almost certainly new discoveries in the field will continue to expand the human life span, and it is not unlikely that there will be some huge breakthroughs as well.

Telomeres And Telomerase

One area of research that holds great promise in extending the human life span lies in the area dealing with telomeres and telomerase.

We saw earlier that, for the most part, the cells of the body have the capacity to divide only a set number of times. Once they reach that limit - the Hayflick limit - and cannot divide further, they lapse into senescence and eventual death. As this happens with more and more cells in the tissues and organs of the body, these organs become increasingly impaired, and less capable of full function. When the failure becomes sufficiently widespread in organs crucial to our existence, we die.

We saw also that this Hayflick limit was tied directly to genetic structures called telomeres. Telomeres, we will recall, are the structures found at the ends of the chromosomes in the nucleus of the cell. The telomeres have been likened to the plastic tips found on the ends of shoelaces. Just as the shoelace tips protect the shoelaces, telomeres protect the chromosomes, particularly when they divide with the cell during cell division.

With each cell division, especially when we are getting on in years, the telomeres grow shorter and shorter. Once they have diminished to a certain critical length, the cell will divide no more.

Telomeres are regulated by an enzyme called telomerase, which is able to direct the telomeres to re-lengthen after each cell division. The ultimate regulator in this causal chain is the telomere gene, which is responsible for the production of telomerase.

As we age, our levels of telomerase decline. This means that there is less telomerase directing the re-lengthening process, which then leads to the consequences we have just looked at: telomeres growing shorter, cells reaching the Hayflick limit and becoming senescent, impending organ failure, and eventual death.

The trick, then, is to step in somewhere along the causal chain and prevent the telomeres from growing shorter.

Some of the research going on today is looking into the regulatory effects that hormones may bring to bear on telomerase production. One study, involving the use of testosterone on stem cells of the rat prostate, has demonstrated that such regulation is possible. Other studies have been looking into the regulatory effects of estrogen on human endometrial cells, These studies, as well, show that regulation of telomerase activity by hormonal means is possible. Another hormone, epidermal growth factor, has shown a strong effect in producing telomerase activity in human epidermal cells. HGH is also thought to hold strong promise in promoting the release of life-lengthening telomerase.

Trials of human telomerase therapy are close to starting at this time for conditions such as cirrhosis of the liver. Dr. Robert Weinberg of MIT's Whitehead Institute says: "To show a connection, you'd want to see that organs are giving out because they've lost telomeres." This has not been proved at this time, but experiments are presently going on in mice.

Most cancer cells produce telomerase to allow themselves to grow forever if nutrition is available. Stopping telomerase production kills the cancer cells. Agents that stop telomerase may be universal chemotherapeutic agents for all tumor types. At this time scientists at Geron Corporation in San Francisco have developed assays to detect telomerase activity and therefore detect cancer. Also, cytotoxic T-cells may be programmed by vaccination to destroy cancer cells that produce excess telomerase. Adenoviruses at this time are also being programmed to enter telomerase producing cancer cells and activate thymidine kinase suicide gene. But how will this help with longevity? The answer is obvious: if we can turn off telomerase production, then we should also be getting close to turning on production of telomerase. Stem cell telomeres are much longer than cancer cell telomeres, and thus should still be intact long after the cancer cells are dead. It may still be a dream to lengthen the telomeres to stop aging, but it is an exciting possibility.

Since telomerase is ultimately under the control of the telomerase gene, much research has been taking place in the genetic aspects of this problem. The range of activity is virtually unlimited: experiments with bacteria, with yeast, with other single celled organisms; experiments on insects, rodents, and humans; and the ever-present statistical analyses.

Some studies done at the University of California by Dr. E. H. Blackburn have involved the use of single celled organisms called ciliates (Tetrahymena thermophila), as well as the yeast, Kluvyeromyces lactis. By causing mutations in the template sequence of telomerase RNA, researchers were ultimately able to show that "...a crucial determinate of telomere length homeostasis is the nature of the duplex DNA--Rap1 protein complex on the very end repeat of the telomere. We propose that this complex plays a complex role in regulating access of telomerase to the telomere." This suggests that it is the molecular makeup at the outer tip of the telomere that plays a large role in the telomere maintaining its length during cell division, adding yet another piece to the puzzle.

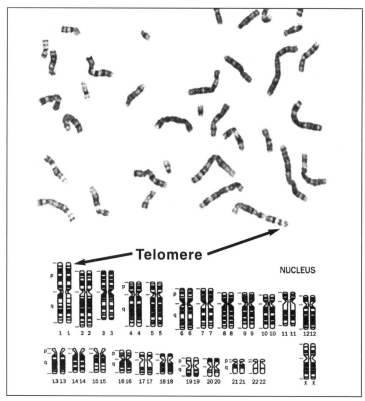

Chromosomes of a human female (22 pairs of Autosomes and 2 sex Chromosomes) The double helix of DNA forms each arm of each chromosome.

At this time in the laboratory, human cells can be kept immortal if telomerase is added. Many cells in our body produce telomerase already. Sperm and egg cells, and some blood and skin cell lines have turned on a production of telomerase. The trick is to now turn on the telomerase gene and allow cells to regenerate throughout the body.

Although the telomere-telomerase research deals with a very complex puzzle, pieces of the puzzle are being solved every day. As further studies continue to provide further solutions to this puzzle, there is little doubt that somewhere in the next decade or two the entire puzzle will be solved. With all the pieces of the puzzle in place, there is also little doubt that it will be accompanied by a huge extension to the human life span. And who knows, perhaps even more.

[Dr. McLeod and Dr. White anticipate with enthusiasm the next symposium on telomerase research.]

Genetics

At the beginning of the 21st Century the initial phase of the Human Genome Project is complete. This means we now have a map of all the genes on all 46 of the human chromosomes. It was a momentous project, and the date of its completion will surely come to be remembered along with other important historical dates

It will likely be some years before this genetic map gives rise directly to practical applications, but give rise to them it surely will. One important thing that the completion of this project does for now is that it signifies and underscores the immense strides being made in the field of genetics today. Further, it foretells of even greater strides that we can expect over the next twenty or thirty years.

We have already seen some of these breakthroughs in the discovery of recombinant HGH, and in the work on mutated telomere genes. The field is abuzz with excitement, and the work important - important because it deals with the basis of all life. Which is why work in genetics often involves so much overlap. Work on any given gene affects whatever that gene is responsible for. And since genetics is at the basis of all life, every discovery in this field invariably has the potential for increasing the human life span.

For example, suppose a particular gene or set of genes was found to predispose an individual to a certain form of cancer. If a method were found in which this gene could be blocked or knocked out, it would have immense implications for the prolonging of human life. And it is discoveries of this sort that we were alluding to earlier, when we said that one of the benefits of maintaining a youthful physiology and remaining in good health, was that you would be around to avail yourself of these future discoveries, and the benefits they will bring.

One discovery in genetics that is already causing a stir involves a gene called MORF-4, short for Mortality Factor from the fourth human chromosome. This gene causes cells to live twice as long as they would normally, and a MORF-4 mutation promotes cell division well beyond its normal limit. Obviously, there are strong possibilities here.

An enzyme called superoxide dismutase enzyme, or SOD, has been used in the past in treating patients for fibrotic scarring after they have undergone radiation treatments. It has also been used to prevent further ongoing damage in heart patients. However, one of the more promising avenues concerning SOD involves the human gene responsible for its production, the SOD-1 gene. This gene has been inserted into the cells of fruit flies. And although the fruit flies make their own SOD, with the addition of the human gene they were able to make even more. Most significantly, they showed a 40% extension to their life span.

Another study on ten rats involved having five of them injected every week with a water solution of DNA and RNA, saturated with chloroform. The five control rats lived out their normal life spans of about 900 days. The injected rats lived anywhere from 1600 to 1900 days, with one of them even living for 2200 days. In human terms, this would represent a life span of about 160 to 220 years. Of course, humans are not rats, but this experiment does point up the fact that there are promising results coming in from a wide variety of studies and experiments.

Some interesting experiments, done in England and completed in August 2000, have shown a doubling in the life span of nematode worms after treatment with superoxide dismutase. (September 7, 2000, Journal of Science)

In a study done on mice, a gene was replaced such that these mice had their life span extended. The important point here is the implication that at least some of the aging process is determined genetically, and that through genetic manipulation, extension to the life span is eminently possible.

Other projects of the future will almost certainly amass data from around the world based on DNA samples from people over 80. This will eventually permit a statistical and demographic analysis that will identify genes that correlate with longevity.

It may take two or three decades before major breakthroughs in genetic research provide ways to take the human life span up to 130 or 150 years. But with all the research going on, breakthroughs are almost certain to show up. In the interim, there will be the less dramatic discoveries unfolding, some of which will inch the life span along a year or two at a time.

The Bolt from the Blue

The history of discovery is replete with accounts of "the bolt from the blue".

In 1896, Henri Bequerel put some photographic plates in a drawer next to some uranium salts. When he retrieved them later he found that the plates had been acted upon as though by some kind of radiation. He had discovered radioactivity.

Another bolt from the blue involved the famed Michelson- Morley experiment, in which the two men measured with great accuracy the speed of light. Up to that time, all velocities were considered to be cumulative. For example, if you were on a train traveling over the earth at 30 miles per hour, and you threw a ball towards the front of the train, the ball would then be traveling over the earth at 60 miles per hour. It was only common sense.

But not so for light. The Michelson-Morley experiment demonstrated that the speed of light is not cumulative, it is constant. If you were to shine a beam of light in the direction of travel, on a train that was moving at 30 miles per hour, the speed of the light beam would not be increased by that 30 miles per hour. The speed of light, regardless of the speed of its source, is always 186,000 miles per second. It is constant. Albert Einstein took this one piece of strange information and from that, produced the revolutionary Special Theory of Relativity. The history of discovery has a number of such stories.

We are certain that the future will bring amazing discoveries in the field of anti-aging, many from the areas we have just looked at. But we are just as certain that there will be discoveries that turn up from extremely unlikely sources, that some of these discoveries will be quite like a bolt from the blue. Because somehow, the pages of history always seem to include them. And these bolts from the blue, along with the expected discoveries, will be there to help you further along the road to longevity.

Immortality

To live forever - that has always been the dream. But in the past, few, if any, have ever really thought it possible, except for the Clan McLeod. As a measure of how prized immortality was we need only consider that most religions posited eternal life as the ultimate end. The trouble was, you had to die to attain it. Whereas: "More time spent in this reality means more time to praise the wonders of God."

Today is different. There is a host of information that separates us from ages past. We know more; we can do more. And some of the things we can do are truly impressive. This has led some people in recent years to contend that immortality is not only possible, it is inevitable. Whether possible, probable, or inevitable, most people today are still quite skeptical. However, it never hurts to keep an open mind.

British poet William Blake wrote: *"What we know now is not the same that it shall be when we know more."*

The meaning inherent in these words is that although we may hold a particular concept at a particular point in time, this concept may well become altered as we come into more information. For instance, at one time the greater part of the human race conceptualized the earth as being flat. But then, as more information accrued, this view of the earth changed. People began to conceptualize the earth as being round. The final piece of information that clinched it was Magellan's circumnavigation of the globe.

The invention of the steam engine also reconfigured our concepts about many things. Prior to the steam engine, the fastest thing around was a horse. The heaviest load that could be hauled was a large wagon, using a team of horses. The introduction of the steam engine changed all that, and today we have the bullet train with speeds approaching 200 miles per hour, and loads in freight trains that run up to 200 cars or more.

Our concepts about flying have also undergone great change. People at one time knew we would never be able to fly through the air, never mind at great speed. Then came the Montgolfier brothers and their hot air balloon, and eventually the Wright brothers with that spindly contraption at Kitty Hawk. And now we have the huge Boeing 747 and the even larger Airbus A380, as well as space shuttles, space stations, and rockets to the moon with tickets to space anticipated from entrepreneurs.

And so it may be in the battle against aging. What we know now will be different when we know more.

There are new advances being made virtually every day: new surgical techniques, new drugs, new treatments, new discoveries. In the past century the average human life span went from about 48 years to where today, in North America, it is now almost 80 years. And climbing all the time.

It is almost certain that the average human life span will climb up to 100, then 130, and eventually to 150 years. It may in time reach 200 years and beyond. And with the advances and discoveries made in the next few decades, and the next century, who can say what the limit is?

To state categorically that immortality is impossible flies in the face of history. So many times in the past, when the majority has decreed something to be impossible, a brave pioneer - an inventor, and explorer, a dreamer - has come forth and demonstrated that this something was possible: the invention was possible; the voyage was possible; the dream was possible.

We cannot say with absolute certainty that we will ultimately attain immortality. That is for the future to decide. But to the cynic who scoffs at the hopes and dreams of others, especially those dreamers who would strive to make the goal of immortality possible, we would say this: "Only those who see the invisible can do the impossible." And we would set forth once more the words of William Blake: "What we know now is not the same that it shall be when we know more."

Because life is precious, we believe it is worth a little effort to extend its time. It is worth a little effort to expand our years.

In reflecting on just how precious life is, we are reminded of the words written by Dylan Thomas. They were written by the poet as his father lay dying, symbolically directed to his father, entreating him to resist mightily the final falling of the curtain. He wrote:

"Do not go gentle into that good night.
Rage, rage against the dying of the light."

Leaving you with these words, we wish you well with whatever program you may embark upon to extend your years. And we hope to see all of you alive and well in the year 2100.

Appendix

Appendix

NOTABLES IN THE FIELD OF ANTI-AGING

Each of us has recognized icons in the field of Longevity Medicine. Dr. Daniel Rudman is well known for his ground breaking research into the benefits of Human Growth Hormone for senior males in an institutional setting published in the New England Journal of Medicine. This publication certainly aroused the interest of many of us and many dived deeper into the field of anti-aging. Dr. Michael Fossel published the book "Reversing Human Aging " in 1996 and suddenly the information was overwhelming. In the early 1990's Dr. Edmund Chein and Dr. Cass Terry of the Medical College of Wisconsin showed in clinical trials that HGH with other balancing of hormones reversed many of the changes of aging. In 1994 Dr. Chein founded the Palm Springs Life Extension Institute and with his large patient base, he has consistently provided invaluable research and observations of his patients. He was a pioneer in using HGH by injection in his practice of medicine and broke new ground for many other physicians following in his footsteps.

Dr. William Rigelson and Carol Colman published "The Superhormone Promise" in 1996. Dr. Rigelson is a leading anti-aging doctor and as a professor of Medicine in Virginia he has helped with the hormone replacement revolution. Another superb author that influenced many health professionals was Dr. John Lee with his book "What Your Doctor May Not Tell You About Menopause." He made inroads for the use of Progesterone in the management of menopause just as Dr. Jerilynn Pryor had proposed in Vancouver B.C. many years before.

Dr. Ron Klatz and Dr. Robert Goldman have been powerhouses in the organization of the anti-aging physicians into the American Academy of Anti Aging Medicine (A4M) and have done much to promote the field to the public at large. There have been many other notable authors that have contributed such as Dr. Eugene Shippen of "The Testosterone Syndrome" and Dr. James Balch of "the Super Antioxidants".

Dr. Philip White and Dr. Don McLeod were instrumental in organizing the first longevity medicine conference in Canada in May 2001, through the Canadian Longevity And Anti Aging Academy (CLA4).

Amino acids 1

The fundamental units of proteins

Amino group (- NH2), carboxyl group (- COOH), H and side chain.

L-Amino acids used by the body.

Amphoteric molecules	i.e. they have both basic and acidic groups
	-electrically neutral
Zwitterions	i.e. at low pH molecule is + ve
	& at high pH molecule is - ve
Essential amino acids	-not made in the body (9)
Conditionally essential	-when inadequate supply (4)
Free form amino acids	-not bound to protein molecule
	-no longer held by electrical charge
	-absorbed in 1/10 of time: (30 mins)
	-goes to directly nourish cells
	-least allergenic
	-act at brain level to increase HGH release
	-act at cell level to promote protein synthesis
Polypeptides	-chains of amino acids
	-may not be absorbed intact (will be at least partly broken down into Amino acids).

Amino acids 2 ~(uptake)

Amino acid uptake multiple pathways:
>   -small neutral amino acids
>   -large neutral and aromatic amino acids
>   -acidic amino acids
>   -basic and cystine
>   -amino acids and glycine
>   -active and passive uptake
>   -2% absorbed in stomach
>   -most uptake in acid pH (upper gut 3.5 - 7.0)
>   -bind in pairs with minerals

Complex Saccharides	-a glucose curve effect.
	-glycosylation pushes amino acid into cells and blood.
Kelp	-provides ions for cell pumps
Collagen	-NASA studies - rabbits could eat 4x more without wt gain

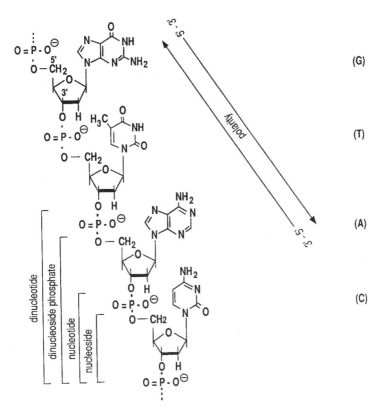

Polarity, Chemical linkages and nomenclature of a portion of DNA

Steroid production in the Ovaries.

The Cholesterol Molecule

Basic four rings of the Steroid molecule.

progesterone   corticosterone   estrone

The basic four ring structure remains the same with only slight variations creating hundreds of possible Steroid molecules.

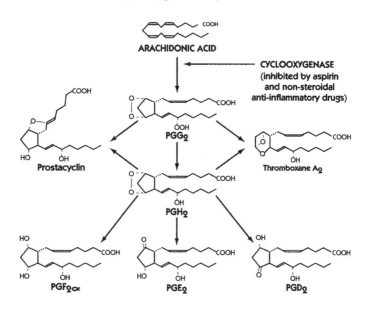

Prostaglandin production from Arachidonic Acid

	FORMULA	NAME
Formula type	Purine bases	

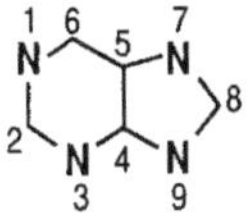

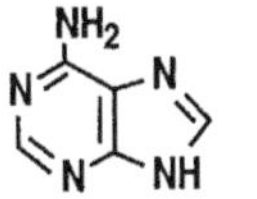

adenine (A)

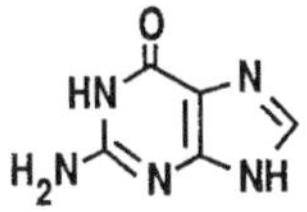

guanine (G)

| | Pyrimidine bases | |

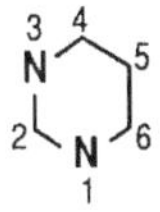

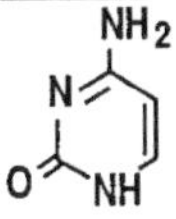

cytosine (C)

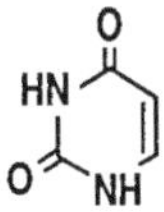

uracil (U)
(in RNA)

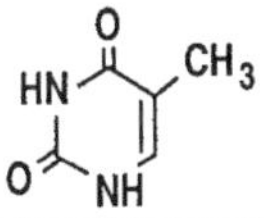

thymine (T)

| | Sugar | |

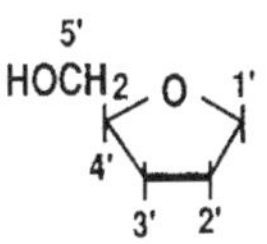

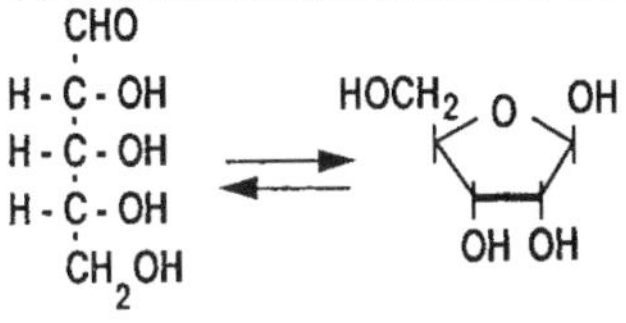

β–D-ribose
(in RNA)

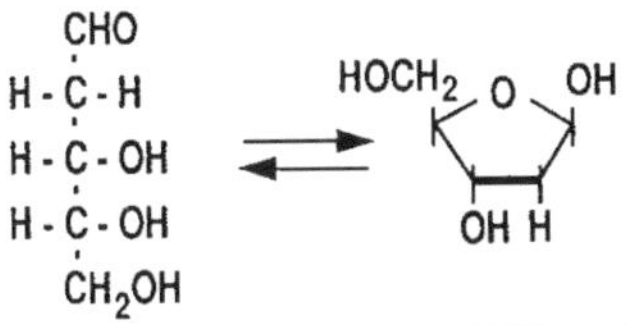

β–2'– deoxyribose
(in DNA)

Amino Acid bases and the (5 Carbon) sugars found in DNA

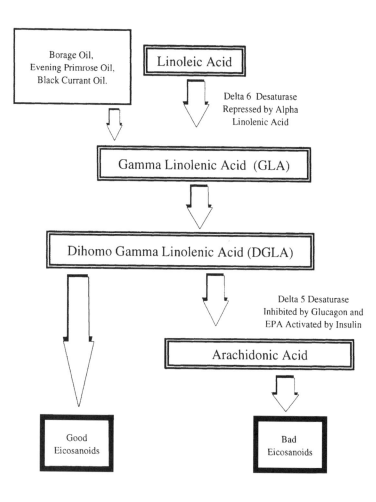

Production of Eicosanoids (short acting local cellular hormones)

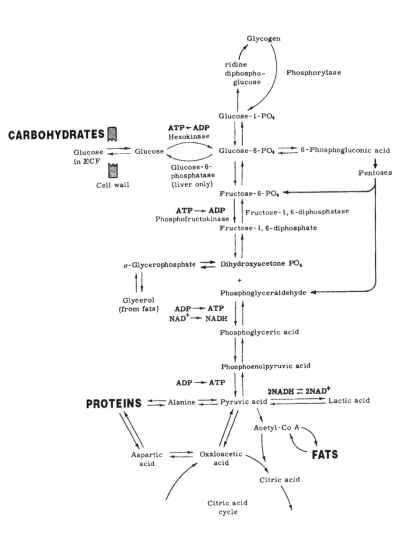

*Enzymes involved in energy production via ATP
from **various food groups**.*

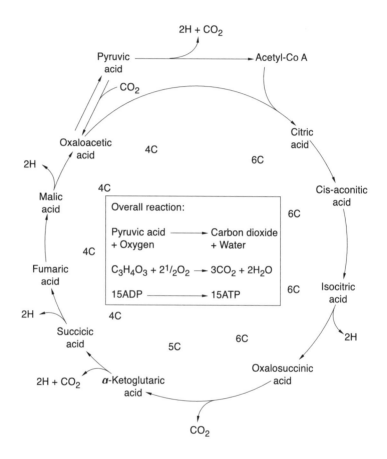

Citric Acid Cycle
for Human energy production

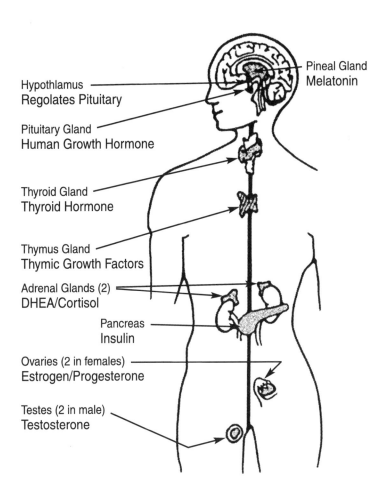

Important Longevity Hormone Production from Organs.

World's Oldest Woman Dies

LONDON - Eva Morris, the world's oldest woman who attributed her longevity to whisky and boiled onions, died in November 2000 - six days short of her 115th birthday. Morris died peacefully in her sleep at a nursing home in the central England town of Stone.

Morris was recognized as the "world's oldest woman" in the Guinness Book of Records.

A former domestic servant who was born in Newcastle-under-Lyme in 1885, Morris was widowed in the 1930's. She lived in her own flat until she was 107, when she moved to the nursing home after a chest infection.

She rode a bicycle, and never had a day's illness apart from occasional chest infections.

Guinness could not immediately confirm who it will now list as the world's oldest woman.

A Dominican, Elizabeth Israel, says she is 125 years old, but does not have the documents to prove it, a Guinness spokesman said.

The oldest man in the world is 111 year old Benjamin Holcomb of Kansas. The oldest person ever with authenticated records was Jeanne Calment of France, who died Aug. 4, 1997, at age 122.

On June 14, Maria do Como Jeronimo, a former slave whose lack of a birth certificate prevented her recognition as the world's oldest woman, died in Itajuba, Brazil. Church records listed her age as 129.

GLYCEMIC INDEX OF CARBOHYDRATES

AVOID RAPID INDUCERS OF INSULIN
GLYCEMIC INDEX MORE THAN 100%

-GRAIN BASED FOODS
   PUFFED RICE
   CORN FLAKES
   PUFFED WHEAT
   MILLET
   INSTANT RICE
   INSTANT POTATO
   FRENCH BREAD
-SIMPLE SUGARS
   MALTOSE
   GLUCOSE
-SNACKS
   TOFU ICE CREAM
   PUFFED RICE CAKES

GLYCEMIC INDEX STANDARD
   = 100 % = WHITE BREAD

GLYCEMIC INDEX 80-100 %

-GRAIN BASED FOODS
   GRAPENUTS
   WHOLEWHEAT BREAD
   ROLLED OATS, OAT BRAN
   MASHED POTATOES
   SLOW WHITE RICE
   BROWN RICE, MUESLI
   SHREDDED WHEAT
-VEGETABLES
   CARROTS, BROAD BEANS
   PARSNIPS, TURNIPS
   CORN, POTATO, BEETS
-FRUITS
   BANANA, PRUNES
   RAISINS, DATES
   APRICOTS, PINEAPPLE
   PAPAYA, MANGO
-SNACKS
   ICE CREAM (LOW-FAT)
   CORN CHIPS, LOWFAT POTATO
   CHIPS, RYE CRISPS
   SPONGE CAKE
-SIMPLE SUGAR
   SUCROSE, CORN SYRUP

---

*HIGH FAT CONTENT RETARDS CARB ABSORPTION INTO THE BODY

MODERATE INDUCERS OF INSULIN

GLYCEMIC INDEX 50 - 80 %

-GRAIN BASED FOODS
   SPAGETTI –REG.+ WHOLE WHEAT
   MOST PASTAS, PITA
   PUMPERNICKEL, ALL-BRAN
                     -FRUITS
   ORANGES AND JUICE
   NON-SWEETENED, LIMES
-VEGETABLES
   PEAS, YAMS, BROCCOLI
   PINTO, GARBANZO BEANS
   KIDNEY, BAKED, NAVY BEANS
-SIMPLE SUGARS
   LACTOSE
-SNACKS
   CANDY BAR* (with FAT)
   POTATO CHIPS WITH FAT*

THE BEST CARBS
REDUCED INSULIN SECRETION
GLYCEMIC INDEX 30 - 50 %

-GRAIN BASED FOODS
   BARLEY
   OATMEAT SLOW COOKING
   WHOLEGRAIN RYEBREAD
-FRUITS
   APPLE, APPLE JUICE
   APPLESAUCE
   PEARS, GRAPES,
   PEACHES, BERRIES
-VEGETABLES
   LENTILS, SPINACH
   LIMA BEANS, PEPPERS
   TOMATO + SOUP
   CHICK PEAS, KALE
-DAIRY PRODUCT
   ICE CREAM HIGH FAT*
   MILK SKIM & WHOLE
   YOGURT, SOUR CREAM

GLYCEMIC INDEX 30 % OR LESS
THE ULTIMATE CARBS
-FRUITS
   CHERRIES and BERRIES
   PLUMS, GRAPEFRUIT
-SIMPLE SUGAR
   FRUCTOSE, MANNITOL
-VEGETABLE -SOY BEANS*
-SNACKS - PEANUTS*

References & Bibliography

References & Bibliography

Section I: Introduction

Brody, J. "Restoring Ebbing Hormones May Slow Aging." *The New York Times,* July 18, 1995.

Chein, E. *"Age Reversal: From Hormones to Telomeres."* Pre-publication proof Wordlink Medical Publishing.

Hayflick, L. *How and Why We Age.* New York: Ballantine Books, 1996.

Kent, S. *The Life Extension Revolution.* New York: Quill, 1980.

Klatz, R., and Kahn, C. Grow *Young With HGH.* HarperCollins, 1997.

Klatz, R.M., ed. *Advances in Anti-Aging Medicine*, vol. 1. New York: Mary Ann Liebert, 1996.

Kolata, G. "New Era of Robust Elderly Belies the Fears of Scientists." *New York Times*, February 27, 1996.

Lawren, "The Hormone that Makes Your Body 20 Years Younger," *Longevity*, October, 1990 p. 34.

Lehrman, Sally "The Fountain of Youth?", *Harvard Health letter*, June 1992 Vol. 17, No. 8. p. 1 (3).

Section II: Aging

Bjorksten, J., "Crosslinkage and the Aging Process," In Rockstein, M. (ed) *Theoretical Aspects of Aging*, Academic Press, New York, 1974, p. 43.

Bjorksten, J., "The Crosslinkage Theory of Aging: Clinical Implications." *Compr Ther* II:65, 1976.

Bryan, T.M., and R.R. Reddel. "Telomere Dynamics and Telomerase Activity in inVitro Immortalised Human Cells." *Eur J Cancer* 33(5):767-773, April 1997.

Campanelli, Linda, C., Ph.D., "Theories of aging," *Theories and Psychosocial Aspects of Aging.* (1) 3-13.

Chang, E., and C.B. Harley. "Telomere Length and Replicative Aging in Human Vascular Tissues." *Proceedings of the National Academy of Sciences* USA 90 (1995): 11190-94.

DaCosta, A.D. "Moderate Caloric Restriction Increases Type 1 IGF Receptors and Protein Synthesis in Aging Rats." *Mechanisms of Ageing Development* 71 (1993): 59-71.

Dilman, V.M. *The Grand Biological Clock.* Moscow: Mir, 1989.

Finch, Caleb, E., *Longevity, Senescence, and the Genome*, University of Chicago Press, 1990.

Harmon, D. *"The Aging Process: Major Risk Factor for Disease and Death." Proceedings of the National Academy of Sciences USA* 88 (June 1991): 5360-5363.

Hayflick, L. *"The Limited In Vitro Lifetime of Human Diploid Cell Strains."* Experimental Cell Research 37 (1965): 614-36.

Hayflick, L.,*How and Why We Age.* New York: Ballantine Books, 1996.

Hayflick, L., "Theories of Aging," in Cape, R., Coe, R., and Rodstein, M. (eds), *Fundamentals of Geriatric Medicine*, Raven Press, New York, 1983.

Kotulak, Ronald, and Gorner, Peter, "Calorie Restriction: Taking the life span to its limit," *Aging on Hold.* Tribune Publishing, 1992, pp. 52-57.

Martin, G.M., Sprague, C.A. and Epstein, C.J., "Replicative Lifespan of Cultivated Human Cells," Lab Invest 23: 26, 1970. *Review of Biological Research in Aging*, Vol. 4, edited by Martin Rothstein, Wiley-Liss, 1990.

Rose, Michael R., *Evolutionary Biology of Aging*, Oxford University Press, 1991.

Rosenfeld, Albert, *Prolongevity II*, Alfred A. Knopf, Inc., New York, 1985, 247-267.

Sharma, Ramesh, "Theories of aging," *Physiological Basis of Aging and Geriatrics*, CRC Press, Florida, 1994, 37-44.

Sonneborn, T., "The Origin, Evolution, Nature, and Causes of Aging," In Behnke, J., Fince, C., and Moment, G. (eds), *The Biology of Aging*, Plenum Press, New York, 1979, p. 341.

Warner, H.R., Butler R.N., Sprott, R.C., and Schneider, E.L., *Modern Biological Theories of Aging*, Raven Press, 1987

Section III: HGH: The Master Hormone

Alba-Roth, J., O.A. Muller, J. Schopohl, et al. "Arginine Stimulates Growth Hormone Secretion By Suppressing Endogenous Somatostatin Secretion." *Journal of Clinical Endocrinology and Metabolism* 67, no. 6 (1988): 1186-89.

Altman, L.K. "Powerful Response Reported to a Combined AIDS Therapy." *New York Times*, July 11, 1996.

Amato, G., G. Izzo, G. LaMontagna, and A. Bellastellal. "Low Dose Recombinant Human Growth Hormone Normalizes Bone Metabolism and Cortical Bone Density and Improves Trabecular Bone Density in Growth Hormone Deficient Adults Without Causing Adverse Effects." *Clinical Endocrinology* (Oxf) 45 (July 1996): 27-32.

Angelin, G. and M. Rudling. "Growth Hormone and Lipoprotein Metabolism." *Endocrinology and Metabolism* 2, suppl. B (1995): 25-28.

Astrom, C., and J. Lindholm. "Growth Hormone-Deficient Young Adults Have Decreased Deep Sleep." *Neuroendocrinology* 51:82-84, January 1990.

Astrom, C., S.A. Pedersen, and J. Lindholm. "The Influence of Growth Hormone On Sleep in Adults With Growth Hormone Deficiency." *Clin Endocrinol (Oxf)* 33:495-500, October 1990.

Bak, B., P.G. Jorgensen, and T.T. Andreassen. "The Stimulating Effect of Growth Hormone on Fracture Healing I Dependent on Onset and Duration of Administration." *Clinical Orthopedics* 264, March 1991: 295-301.

Bansch, D., et al. "Basal Growth Hormone Levels are Positively Correlated with High Density Lipoprotein Cholesterol Levels in Women." *Metabolism* 46, No. 9 (1997): 1039-43.

Bar-Dayan, Y., and M. Small. "Effect of Bovine Growth Hormone Administration on the Pattern of Thymic Involution in Mice." *Thymus* 23, no. 2 (1994): 95-101.

Beaubien, G. "Why Get Old?" *Chicago Tribune*. October 20, 1994.

Bengtssön, B-A, et al. "Treatment of Adults with Growth Hormone (GH) Deficiency with Recombinant Human GH." *Journal of Clinical Indocrinology and Metabolism* 76 (1993): 309-17.

Bengtssön, B-A. "The Consequences of Growth Hormone Deficiency in Adults." *Acta Endocrinologica* 128, suppl. 2(1993): 2-5.

Bengtssön, B-A., et al. "Cardiovascular Risk Factors in Adults with Growth Hormone Deficiency." *Endocrinology and Metabolism* 2, suppl. B (1995): 29-35.

Bengtssön, B-A. *An Introduction to Growth Hormone Deficiency in Adults*. Oxford, England: Oxford Clinical Communications, 1993

Bengtssön, B-A. "Effects of Bone Mineral Content; Stimulation of Bone and Cartilage Growth." Submitted for publication.

Beshyah, S. A. "The Effects of Short and Long Term Growth Hormone Replacement Therapy in Hypopituitary Adults on Lipid Metabolism and Carbohydrate Tolerance." *Journal of Clinical Endocrinology and Metabolism* 80 (1995): 356-63.

Bianda, T., Y. Gatz, R. Bouillon, E.R. Froesch, and C. Schmid. "Effects of Short-Term Insulin-Like Growth Factor-1 (IGF-1) or Growth

Hormone (GH) Treatment on Bone Metabolism and on Production of 1,25-dihydroxycholecalciferol in GH- Deficient Adults." *J Clin Endocrinol Metab* 83(1):81-87, January 1998.

Bier, S.M. "Growth Hormone and Insulin-Like Growth Factor 1: Nutritional Pathophysiology and Therapeutic Potential." Acta-*Paediatr.-Scand.-Suppl.* 374 (1991): 119-28.

Binnerts, A., G.R. Swart, J.H. Wilson, N. Googebrugger, H.A. Pols, J.C. Birkenhager, and S.Wl Lamberts. "The Effect of Growth Hormone Administration in Growth Hormone Deficient Adults on Bone Protein, Carbohydrate and Lipid Homeo-stasis, As Well As On Body Composition." *Clin Endocrinol* (Oxf) 37:79-87, July 1992.

Bjarnason, R., R. Wickelgren, M. Hermansson, F. Hammarqvist, B. Carlsson, and L.M. Carlsson. "Growth Hormone Treatment Prevents the Decrease in Insulin-Like Growth Factor 1 Gene Expression in Patients Undergoing Abdominal Surgery. *Journal of Clinical Endocrinology and Metabolism* 83(5) (May 1998): 1566-1572.

Bjorntorp, P. "Neuroendocrine Ageing." *Journal of Internal Medicine* 238, no. 5 (November 1995): 401-04.

Borst, J.E., et al. "Studies of GH Secretagogues in Man." *Journal of the American Geriatrics Society* 42, no. 5 (May 1995): 532-4.

Bouillon, R. "*Growth Hormone and Bone.*" Horm Res 36 Suppl. 1:49-55, 1991.

Brixen, K., et al. "Growth Hormone (GH) and Adult Bone Remodeling: The Potential Use of GH in Treatment of Osteoporosis." *Journal of Pediatric Endocrinology* (England) 6, no. 1 (January-March 1993): 65-71.

Brixen, K., M. Dassem, H>D. Nielsen, A.G. Loft, A. Flyvbjerg, and L. Mosekilde. "Short-Term Treatment With Growth Hormone Stimulates Osteoblastic and Osteoclastic Activity in Osteopenic Postmenopausal Women: A Dose Response Study." *J Bone Miner Res* 10(12): 1865-1874, December 1995.

Brody, J. "Restoring Ebbing Hormones May Slow Aging." *The New York Times* B5-6. 18 July 1995.

Brownlee, S., and T. Watson. Can a Hormone Fight AIDS? (Human Growth Hormone)." *U.S. News & World Report*, November 21 1994.

Caidahl, K., S. Eden, and B-A. Bengtssön. "Cardiovascular and Renal Effects of Growth Hormone, Clinical Endocrinology (Oxford, England) 40, no. 3 (March 1994): 393-400.

Capaldo, B., G. Lembo, V. Rendina, C. Vigorito, R. Guida, A. Cuocolo, S. Fazio, and L. Sacca. "Sympathetic Deactivation by Growth Hormone Treatment in Patients With Dilated Cardiomyopathy." *Eur Heart J* 19(4): 623-627, April 1998.

Casanueva, F.F., L. Villaneuva, J.A. Cabranes, et al. "Cholinergic Mediation of Growth Hormone Secretion Elicited by Arginine, Clondine, and Physical Exercise in Man." *Journal of Coinical Endocrinology and Metabolism* 52, no. 3 (March 1981): 409-15.

Cash, C.D. "Gammahydroxybutyrate: An Overview of the Pros and Cons for It Being a Neurotransmitter And/Or a Useful Therapeutic Agent." *Neuroscience and Biobehavioral Reviews* 18, no. 2 (1994): 291-304.

Cella, S.G., Valerio Moiraghi, Francesco Minuto, et al. "Prolonged Fasting or Clonidine Can Restore the Defective Growth Hormone Secretion in Old Dogs." *Acta Endocrinologica* (Copenhagen) 121, no. 2 (1989):177-84.

Chaney, M.M. "The Effect of Oral Arginine, Age, and Exercise on Growth Hormone, Insulin, and Blood Glucose." *Dissertation Abstracts International* 50, no. 10 (April 1990).

Cheek, D.B., and D.E. Hill. "Effects of Growth Hormone on Cell and Somatic Growth."
    in *Handbook of Physiology: A Critical Comprehensive Presentation of Physiological Knowledge and Concepts -Section 7:2: Endocrinology-Part 1*:
        Female Reproductive System. R.O. Greep and E.B. Astwood, eds. Washington: American Physiological Society, 4(7):159-185, 1973.

Chein, E. "*Age Reversal: From Hormones to Telomeres.* Pre-Publication Proof. Wordlink Medical Publishing.

Christ, E.R., P.V. Carroll, D.L. Russel-Jones, and P.H. Sonksen. "The Consequences of Growth Hormone Deficiency in Adulthood, and the Effects of Growth Hormone Replacement. *Schweiz Med Wochenschr* 127(35): 1440-1449, 30 August 1992.

Christensen, H., H. Oxlund, and S. Laurberg. "Postoperative Biosynthetic Human Growth Hormone Increases the Strength and Collagen Deposition of Experimental Colonic Anastomoses." *International Journal of Colorectal Diseases* 6, no. 3 (August 1991): 133-38.

Christensen H., A. Flyvbjerg, H. Orskov, and S. Laurberg. "Effects of Growth Hormone on the Inflammatory Activity of Experimental Colitis in Rats." *Scand J Gastroenterol* 28(6):503-511, June 1993.

Christiansen, J.S., et al. "Effects of Growth Hormone on Body Composition in Adults." *Hormone Research* 33, suppl. 4 (1990): 61-64

Christiansen, J.S., et al. "GH-Replacement Therapy in Adults." *Hormone Research* 36, suppl. 1 (1991): 66-72.

Clemmons, D.R., and L.E. Underwood. "Growth Hormone As a Potential Adjunctive Therapy for Weight Loss." In Human Growth *Hormone: Progress and Challenges,* edited by L.E. Underwood. New York: Marcel Dekker, 1986.

Cole, B.R. "Recombinant Human Growth Hormone Therapy in Renal Insufficiency: New Hope for Children" (editorial). *Journal of the American Society of Nephrology* 1, no. 10 (April 1991): 1127.

Conteras, V. "Natural Method for Boosting Human Growth Hormone." *Journal of Longevity Research* 1, no. 8 (1995): 38-39.

Cordido, F., et al. "Massive Growth Hormone Discharge in Obese Subjects After the Combined Administration of GH-Releasing Hormone and GHRP-6: Evidence for a Marked Somatroph Secretory Capability in Obesity." *Journal of Clinical Endocrinology and Metabolism* 76 (1983): 819-23.

Corpas, E., S.M. Harman, and M.R. Blackman. "*Human Growth Hormone and Human Aging*." Endocrine Reviews 14, no. 1 (1993): 20-39.

Crist, D.M. et al. "Exogenous Growth Hormone Treatment Alters Body Composition and Increases Natural Killer Cell Activity in Women with Impaired Endogenous Growth Hormone Secretion." *Metabolism* 36, no. 12 (1987):   1115-17.

Crist, D.M., Peake, G.T., Egan, P.A., Waters, D.L., "Body Composition Response to Exogenous GH during Training in Highly Conditioned Adults." *Journal of Applied Physiology* 65 1988: 579-584.

Cuneo, R.C., et al. "Cardiac Failure Responding to Growth Hormone." *Lancet*, April 15, 1989: 838-9.

Cuneo, R.C. et al. "Cardiovascular Effects of Growth Hormone Treatment in Growth-   Hormone-Deficient Adults: Stimulation of the Renin-Aldosterone System." *Clinical Sciences* 81, no. 5 (November 1991): 587-92.

Cuneo, R.C. et al. "Diagnosis of Growth Hormone Deficiency." *Clinical Endocrinology* 37 (1992): 387-97.

Cuneo, R.C., F. Salomon, C.M. Wiles, R. Hesp, and P.H. Sonksen. "Growth Hormone Treatment in Growth Hormone-Deficient Adults: I. Effects on Muscle Mass and Strength." *J Appl Physiol* 70:688-694, February 1991.

Cuneo, R.C., F. Salomon, C.M. Wiles, R. Hesp, and P.H. Sonksen. "Growth Hormone Treatment in Growth Hormone-Deficient Adults: II. Effects On Exercise Performance." *J Appl Physiol* 70:695-700, February 1991.

Daubeney, P.E.F., et al. "Cardiac Effects of Growth Hormone in Short Normal Children: Results After Four Years of Treatment." *Archives of Disease in Childhood* 72 (1993): 337-39.

Daughaday, W.H. and S. Harvey. "Growth Hormone Action: Clinical Significance." In *Growth Hormone*, edited by S. Harvey, C.G. Scanes, and W.H. Daughaday. Boca Raton, Fla.: CRC Press, Boca Raton, 1995.

Davila, D.R. et al. "Role of Growth Hormone in Regulating T-Dependent Immune Events in Aged, Nude, and Transgenic Rodents." *Journal of Neuroscience Research* 18 (1987): 108-16.

Dean, W. *Biological Aging Measurement: Clinical Applications*. Los Angeles: The Center for Bio-Gerontology, 1988.

De Boer, H., et al. "Diagnosis of Growth Hormone Deficiency in Adults." *Lancet* 343 (June 25, 1994): 1645-46.

De Boer, H.D. G.J. Blok, and E.A. Van Der Veen. "Clinical Aspects of Growth Hormone Deficiency in Adults." *Endocrine Reviews* 16 no. 1 (1995): 63-86.

DeBoer, H., G.J. Blok, B. Voerman, P. Derriks, and E. van der Veen. "Changes in Subcutaneous and Visceral Fat Mass During Growth Hormone Replacement in Adult Men." *Int J Obes Relat Metab Disord* 20(6):580-587, June 1996.

Degerblad,M., et al. "Reduced Bone Mineral Density in Adults with Growth Hormone Deficiency: Increased Bone Turnover During 12 Months of GH Substitution Therapy." European Journal of Endocrinology 133, no. 2 (August 1995): 180-88.

Deijen, J.B., et al. "Cognitive Impairments and Mood Disturbances in Growth Hormone Deficient Men." Manuscript in preparation.

Dilman, V.M. *The Grand Biological Clock*. Moscow: Mir, 1989.

Donaldson, Thomas, Ph.D., *Life Extension Report*, April 1991, Vol. 11, No. 4, p. 32.

Eriksen, E.F., M. Kassem, and K. Brixen. "Growth Hormone and Insulin-Like Growth Factors As Anabolic Therapies for Osteoporosis." *Hormone Research* 40, nos. 1-3   (1993): 95-98.

Erickson, D. "Big-Time Orphan: Human Growth Hormone Could Be a Blockbuster." *Scientific American*, September 1990, 165-66.

Falanga, V. "Growth Factors and Wound Healing." *Dermatologic Clinics* 11, no. 4 (October 1993): 667-675.

Fazio, S. "Preliminary Study of Growth Hormone in the Treatment of Dilated Cardio-myopathy." *New England Journal of Medicine* 334 (March 28, 1996): 809-14.

Frustaci, A., et al. "Reversible Dilated Cardiomyopathy Due to Growth Hormone Deficiency." *American Journal of Clinical Pathology* 97 (1992): 503-11.

Fujita K., H. Terada, and L.Z. Ling. "Male Sexual Insufficiency." *Nippon Rinsho* 55(11): 2908-2913, November 1997.

Greenspan, Francis S., Baxter, John D.   "Basic & Clinical Endocrinology." Lange Medical Book, Fourth Edition.

Giampapa, V.C., R.M. Klatz, B.E. Di Bernardo, and F.A. Kovarik. "Biomarker Matrix Protocol." *In Advances in Anti-Aging Medicine,* vol. 1, edited by R.M. Klatz. New York: Mary Ann Liebert, 1996.

Gluckman, P., N. Klempt, J. Guan, C. Mallard, I. Sirimanne, M. Dragunow, M. Klempt, K. Singh, C. Williams, and K. Nikolics. "A Role For IGF-1 in the Rescue of CNS Neurons Following Hypoxic-Ischemic Injury." *Biochem Biophys Res Commun* 182(2): 593-599, January 1992.

Goff, B.L. et al. "Growth Hormone Treatment Stimulates Thymulin Production in Aged Dogs." *Clinical and Experimental Immunology* 68 (1987): 580-97.

Gottardis, M., A. Benzer, W. Koller, T.J. Luger, F. Puhringer, and J. Hackl. "Improvement in Septic Syndrome After Administration of Recombinant Human Growth Hormone (rhGh)." *Journal of Trauma* 31, no. 1 (January 1991): 81-86.

Goya, R.G., M.C. Gagnerault, M.C. DeMoraes, W. Savino, and M. Dardeen. "In Vivo Effects of Growth Hormone on Thymus Function in Aging Mice." *Brain Behav. Immun.* 6, no. 4 (December 1992): 341-54.

Grinspoon, S.K., H.B. Baum, S. Peterson, and A. Klibanski. "Effects of rhIGF-1 Administration on Bone Turnover During Short-Term Fasting." *J Clin Invest* 96(2):900-906, August 1995.

Harvey, S. "Growth Hormone Action: Neural Function." In Growth Hormone, edited by S. Harvey, C.G. Scanes, and W.H. Daughaday. Boca Raton, Fla.: CRC Press, Boca Raton, 1995.

Harvey, S., C.G. Scanes, and W.H. Daughaday, eds. *Growth Hormone.* Boca Raton, Fla.: CRC Press, 1995.

Hayflick, L. *How and Why We Age.* New York: Ballantine Books, 1996.

Hendler, S.S. The Doctors' Vitamin and Mineral Encyclopedia. New York City: Simon & Schuster, 1990.

Hertoghe, T. "Growth Hormone Therapy in Aging Adults: Place and Dosage in a Multiple Hormonal Replacement Therapy.: 1996 European Congress on Anti-Aging Medicine, Madrid, Spain.

Hesse, V., et al. "Insulin-Like Growth Factor I Correlations to Changes of the Hormonal Status in Puberty and Age." *Experimental and Clinical Endocrinology* 102, no. 4 (1994): 289-98.

Hirschberg, R. "Effects of Growth Hormone and IGF-1 On Glomerular Ultra Filtration in Growth Hormone-Deficient Rats." *Regul Pept* 48(1-2):241-250, October 1993.

Ho, K.Y., and A.J. Weussberger. "The Antinatriuretic Action of Biosynthetic Human Growth Hormone in Man Involves Activation of the Renin-Angiotensin System." *Metabolism* 39 (1990): 133-37.

Hodes, R.J. "Frailty and Disability: Can Growth Hormone or Other Trophic Agents Make a Difference?" *Journal of the American Geriatric Society* 42 (1994): 1208-11.

Hoffman, A.R., et al. "Growth Hormone Therapy in the Elderly: Implications for the Aging Brain." *Psychoneuroimmunology* 17, no. 4 (1992): 327-333.

Hoffman, D.M., et al. "Diagnosis of Growth-Hormone Deficiency in Adults." *Lancet* 343 (1994):1064-68.

Howard, Ben, "Growing Younger.." *Longevity*. October, 1992: p.41.

Hwu, C.M., C.F. Kwok, T.Y. Lai, K.C. Lee, L.C. Hsiao, S.H. Lee, V.S. Fang, and L.T. Ho. "Growth Hormone (GH) Replacement Reduces Total Body Fat and Normalizes Insulin Sensitivity in GH-Deficient Adults: A Report of One-Year Clinical Experience." *J Clin Endocrinol Metab* 82(10): 3285-3292, October 1997.

Iannoli P., J.H. Miller, C.K. Ryan, L.G. Gu, T.R. Ziegler, and H.C. Sax. "Epidermal Growth Factor and Human Growth Hormone Accelerate Adaptation After Massive Enterectomy in an Additive, Nutrient-Dependent, and Site-Specific Fashion." *Surgery* 122(4):721-728, October 2997.

Imagawa, S., M.A. Goldberg, J. Doweiko, and H.G. Bunn. "Regulatory Elements of the Erythropoietin Gene." *Blood* 77, no. 2(January 1991): 278-85.

Inzucchi, S.E., and R.J. Robbins. "Effects of Growth Hormone on Human on Human Bone Biology." *Journal of Clinical Endocrinology and Metabolism* 79, no. 3 (1994): 691-94.

Iranmanesh, A., G. Lizarralde, and J.D. Veldhuis. "Age and Relative Adiposity Are Specific Negative Determinants of the Frequency and Amplitude of Growth Hormone (GH) Secretory Bursts and the Half-Life of Endogenous GH in Healthy Men." *Journal of Clinical Endocrinology and Metabolism* 73 (1991): 1081-88.

Isadori, A., A.L. Monaco, M. Cappa, et al. "A Study of Growth Hormone Release in Man After Oral Administration of Amino Acids." *Current Medical Research and Opinion* 7, no. 7 (1981): 475-81.

James, J.S. "Human Growth Hormone Reverses Wasting in Clinical Trial." AIDS Treatment News, August 19, 1994. Jardieu, P., R. Clark, D. Mortensen, and K. Dorshkind. "In Vivo Administration of Insulin-Like Growth-Factor-1 Stimulates Primary B Lymphopoiesis and Enhances Lumphocyte Recovery After Bone Marrow Transplantation." *J Immunol* 152(9): 4320-4327, May 1994.

Johansson, A.G., P.Burman, K. Westermark, and S. Ljunghall. "The Bone Mineral   Density in Acquired Growth Hormone Deficiency Correlates With Circulating Levels of Insulin-Like Growth Factor 1." *J Intern Med* 232:447-452, November 1992.

Johannson, G., et al. "Growth Hormone Treatment of Abdominally Obese Men Reduces Abdominal Fat Mass, Improves Glucose and Lipoprotein Metabolism and Reduces Diastolic Blood Pressure." *Journal of Clinical Endocrinology and Metabolism* 82 (1997): 727-34.

Johannson, G., et al. "Two Years of Growth Hormone (GH) Treatment Increase Isometric and Isokinetic Muscle Strength in GH-Deficient Adults." *Journal of Clinical Endocrinology and Metabolism* 82 (1997): 2877-84.

Johannsson, G., T. Rosen, I. Bosaeus, L. Sjorstrom, and B-A Bengtssön. "Two Years of Growth Hormone Treatment in Growth-Hormone-Deficient Adults Normalised Body Composition and Induced Favourable Changes in Cardiovascular Risk Factors." In press.

Johannsson, G., T. Rosen, I. Bosaeus, L. Sjorstrom, and B-A. Bengtssön. "Two Years of Growth Hormone Treatment Increases Bone Mineral Content and Density in Hypopituitary Patients with Adult-Onset Growth Hormone Deficiency." *Journal of Clinical Endocrinology and Metabolism* 81, no. 8 (1996):2865-73.

Johannsson, J.O., G. Larson, M. Andersson, A. Elmgren, L. Hynsjo, A. Lindahl, P.A. Lundberg, O.G.P. Isaksson, S. Lindstedt, and B-A. Bengtssön. "Treatment of Growth Hormone-Deficient Adults with Recombinant Human Growth Hormone Increases the Concentration of Growth Hormone in the Cerebrospinal Fluids and Affects Neurotransmitters." *Neuroencocrinology* 61 (1995): 57-66.

Johannsson, J.O., L. Kerstin, L. Tengborn, T. Rosen and B-A Bengtssön. "High Fibrinogen and Plasminogen Activator Inhibitor Activity in Growth-Hormone-Deficient Adults." Manuscript in preparation.

Johnston, B.M., E.C. Mallard, C.E. Williams, and P.D. Gluckman. "Insulin-Like Growth Factor-1 Is a Potent Neuronal Rescue Agent

After Hypoxic-Ischemic Injury in Fetal Lambs." *Journal of Clinical Investigation* 97, no. 2 (January 15, 1996): 300-08.

Jorgensen, J.O.L. "Adult Growth Hormone Deficiency." *Hormone Research* 42 (1994): 235-41.

Jorgensen, J.O.L., et al. "Three Years of Growth Hormone Treatment in Growth Hormone Deficient Adults: Near Normalization of Body Composition and Physical Performance." *European Journal of Endocrinology* 130 (1994): 224-8.

Jorgensen, J.O., S.A. Pedersen, L. Thuesen, J. Jorgensen, T. Ingemann-Hansen, N.E. Skakkebaek, and J.S. Christiansen. "Beneficial Effects of Growth Hormone Treatment in GH-Deficient Adults." *Lancet* 1:1221-1225, June 1989.

Jospe, N., and K.R. Powell. "Growth Hormone Deficiency in an 8-Year-Old Girl With Human Immunodeficiency Virus Infection." *Pediatrics* 86(2):309-312 August 1990.

Kahn, C. *Beyond the Helix: DNA and the Quest for the Secrets of Aging*. New York: Times Books, 1985.

Kaiser, F.E., A.J. Silver, and JE. Morley. "The Effect of Recombinant Human Growth Hormone on Malnourished Older Individuals." *Journal of the American Geriatrics Society* 39 (1991): 235-40.

Kaplan, S. L. "The Newer Uses of Growth Hormone in Adults." *Advances in Internal Medicine* 38 (1993): 387 ff.

Kasai, K. M. Kobayashi, and S. Shimoda. "Stimulatory Effects of Oral Glycine On Human Growth Hormone Secretion." *Metab* 27(2):201-208, February 1978.

Kelley, K.W. "Growth Hormone in Immunobiology." In *Psychoneuroimmunology* 2nd edition, edited by R. Ader, D.L. Feltern, and N. Cohen. New York: Academic Press, 1991.

Kelley, K.W. "Immunologic Roles of Two Metabolic Hormones, Growth Hormone and Insulin-Like Growth Factor-1, in Aged Animals." *Nutritional Reviews* 53, no.4 (1995): S95-S104.

Kelley, K.W., et al. "GH3 Pituitary Adenoma Implants Can Reverse Thymic Aging." *Proceedings of the National Academy of Sciences* USA 83 (1986): 5663-67.

Kelley K.W., et al. "A Pituitary-Thymus Connection During Aging." *Annals of the New York Academy of Sciences* 521 (1988): 88-98.

Khansari, D.N., and T. Gustad. "Effects of Long-Term, Low-Dose Growth Hormone Therapy on Immune Function and Life Expectancy of Mice." *Mechanisms of Ageing and Development* 57 (1991): 87-100.

Kimbrough, T.D., S. Sherman, T.R. Ziegler, M. Scheltinga, and D.W. Wilmore. "Insulin-Like Growth Factor-1 Response Is Comparable Following Intravenous and Subcutaneous Administration of Growth Hormone." *Journal of Surgical Research* 51 (December 1991): 472-76.

Kovaks, G., et al. "Growth Hormone Prevents Steroid-Induced Growth Depression in Health and Uremia." *Kidney Int.* 40 no. 6 (December 1991): 1032-40.

Kraemer, W.J., et al. "Endogenous Anabolic Hormonal and Growth Factor Responses to Heavy Resistance Exercise in Males and Females." *International Journal of Sports Medicine* 12 (1991): 228-35.

Landin-Wilheimsen, et al. "Serum Insulin-Like Growth Factor 1 in a Random Population Sample of Men and Women: Relation to Age, Sex, Smoking Habits, Coffee Consumption and Physical Activity, Blood Pressure, and Concentrations of Plasma Lipids, Fibrinogen, Parathyroid Hormone and Osteocalcin." *Clinical Endocrinology* 41 (1994):351-57.

Laursen, T., J.O. Jorgennsen, and J.S. Christianssen. "Metabolic Effects of Growth Hormone Administered Subcutaneously Once or Twice Daily to Growth Hormone Deficient Adults." *Clin Endocrinol* (Oxf) 41(3):337-343, September 1994.

Lawler, B., et al. "Growth Hormone Treatment Stimulates Thymulin Production in Aged Dogs." *Clinical and Experimental Immunology* 68 (1987): 580-87.

Lawren, "The Hormone that Makes Your Body 20 Years Younger," *Longevity*, October 1990, p. 34.

Lehrman, Sally, "The Fountain of Youth?", *Harvard Health Letter*, June 1992 Vol.17, No. 8, p.1 (3).

Lewin, D.L. "Growth Hormone and Age: Something to Sleep On?" Journal of NIH *Research* 7 (1993):34-35.

Levy, J.B., and D.A. Hussmann. "Micropenis Secondary To Growth Hormone Deficiency: Does Treatment With Growth Hormone Alone Result in Adequate Penile Growth?" *J Urol* 156(1):214-216, July 1996.

Lieberman, S.A., et al. "Anabolic Effects of Recombinant Insulin-Like Growth Factor-1in Cachectic Patients with the Acquired Immunodeficiency Syndrome." *Journal of Clinical Endocrinology and Metabolism* 78, no. 2 (1994): 404-10.

Loh, E., and J.L. Swain. "Growth Hormone for Heart Failure--Cause for Cautious Optimism." *New England Journal of Medicine* 334 (March 28, 1996): 856-57.

Lombardi, G., A. Colao, A. Cuocolo, A. Longobardi, C. DiSomma, F. Orio, B. Merola, E. Nicolai, and M. Salvatore. "Cardiological Aspects of Growth Hormone and Insulin-Like Growth Factor-1." *J Pediatr Endocrinol Metab* 10(6):553-560, November 1997.

Marcus R., Butterfield, Gl, Holloway, L., et al. "Effects of Short-Term Administration of Recombinant Human Growth Hormone to Elderly People," *Journal of Clinical Endocrinology and Metabolism* 1990: 519-27.

Massey, K.A., C. Blakeslee, and H.S. Pitkow. "Possible Therapeutic Effects of Growth Hormone On Wound Healing in the Diabetic Patient." *J Am Podiatr Assoc* 88(1): 25-29, January 1998.

McGauley, G.A., et al. "Psychological Well-Being Before and After Growth Hormone Treatment in Adults with Growth Hormone Deficiency.: *Hormone Research* 33, suppl. 4 (1990): 52-54.

Meling, T.R., and E.S. Nylen. "Growth Hormone Deficiency in Adults: A Review." *Am J Med Sci* 311: 153-166, April 1996.

Mendelson, W.B., S. Slater, P. Gold, and J.C. Gillin. "The Effect of Growth Hormone Administration On Human Sleep: A Dose-Response Study." *Biol Psychiatry* 15:613-616, August 1980.

Merimee, et al., "Arginine Initiated Release of Growth Hormone: Factors Modifying the Response in Normal Men," *New England Journal of Medicine.* 280(26): 1434-38 (1969).

Mulligan, K., C. Grunfeld, M.K. Hellerstein, R.A. Neese, and M. Schambelan. "Anabolic Effects of Recombinant Human Growth Hormone in Patients with Wasting Associated with Human Immunodeficiency Virus Infection." *Journal of Clinical Endocrinology and Metabolism* 77 (1993): 956-62.

Nass, R., R.M. Huber, V. Klauss, O.A. Muller, J. Schopohl, and C.J. Strasburger. "Effect of Growth Hormone Replacement Therapy On Physical Work Capacity and Cardiac and Pulmonary Function in Patients With Growth Hormone Deficiency Acquired in Adulthood." *J Clin Endocrinol Metab* 80:552-557, February 1995.

Nass, R., and C.J. Strasburger. "Effects of Growth Hormone Treatment On Serum Lipids and Lipoproteins in Adults With Growth Hormone Deficiency." *Eur J Endocrinol* 130 Suppl 2:34, 1994.

O'Halloran, D.J., A. Tsatsoulis, R.W. Whitehouse, S.J. Holmes, J.E. Adams, and S.M. Shalet. "Increased Bone Density After Recombinant Human Growth Hormone (GH) Therapy in Adults With Isolated GH Deficiency." *J Clin Endocrinol Metab* 76:1344-1348, May 1993.

Ohlsson, C., et al. "Growth Hormone Induces Multiplation of the Slowly Cycling Germinal Cells of the Rat Tibial Growth Plate." *Proceedings of the National Academy of Science USA* 89 (October 1992): 9826-30.

Orme, S.M. "Comparison of Measures of Body Composition in a Trial of Low Dose Growth Hormone Replacement Therapy." *Clinical Endocrinology* 37 (1992): 453-59.

O'Shea, M., S.B. Miller, K. Finkel, and M.R. Hammerman. "Roles of Growth Hormone and Growth Factors in the Pathogenesis and Treatment of Kidney Disease." *Curr Opin Nephrol Hypertens* 2(1):67-72, January 1993.

Osterziel, K.J., R. Markus, R. Willenbrock, O. Strohm, and R. Dietz. "Therapy of Dilated Cardimyopathy With Recombinant Human Growth Hormone." *Z Kardiol* 86(10):803-811, October 1997.

Ottosson, M., et al. "Growth Hormone Inhibits Lipoprotein Lipase Activity in Human Adipose Tissue." *Journal of Clinical Endocrinology and Metabolism* 80 (1995): 936-41.

Ovesen, P. J.O. Jorgensen, J. Ingerslev, K.K. Ho, H. Orskov, and J.S. Christiansen. "Growth Hormone Treatment of Subfertile Males." *Fertil Steril* 66(2):292-298, August 1996.

Papadakis, M.A. et al. "Growth Hormone Replacement in Healthy Older Men Improves Body Composition But Not Functional Ability." *Annals of Internal Medicine* 124 (1996): 708-16.

Pearson, D., and S. Shaw. *The Life Extension Weight Loss Program.* New York: Doubleday, 1986.

Pearson, D., and S. Shaw. Life Extension: *A Practical Scientific Approach.* New York: Warner Books, 1982.

Perring, M., and J. Moral. "Holistic Approach to the Management of Erectile Disorders in a Male Sexual Health Clinic." *British Journal of Clinical Practice* 49, no. 3 (May-June 1995): 140.

Powrie, J., A. Weissberger, and P. Sonksen. "Growth Hormone Replacement Therapy For Growth Hormone-Deficient Adults." *Drugs* 49(5): 656-663, May 1995.

Raben, M.S. "Treatment of Pituitary Dwarf with Human Growth Hormone." *Journal of Clinical Endocrinology* 18 (1958): 901-03.

Rabinowitz, D., and K.L. Ziebler. "A Metabolic Regulating Device Based on the Actions of Human Growth Hormone and Insulin, Singly and Together, on the Human Forearm." *Nature* 199 (August 31, 1963): 913-15.

Richelsen, B., et al. "Growth Hormone Treatment of Obese Women for 5 Weeks: Effect on Body Composition and Adipose Tissue LPL Activity." *American Journal of Physiology* 226, no.2, pt 1 (1994):E211-16.

Rosen, C.J., et al. "Insulin-Like Growth Factors and Bone: The Osteoporosis Connection." *Proceedings of the Society for Experimental Biology* 206 (1994): 83-102.

Rosen, T., et al. "Cardiovascular Risk Factors in Adult Patients with Growth Hormone Deficiency." *Acta Endocrinologica* 129, no. 3 (September 1993): 195-200.

Rosen, T., et al. "Consequences of Growth Hormone Deficiency in Adults and the Benefits and Risks of Recombinant Human Growth Hormone Treatment." *Hormone Research* 43 (1995): 93-99.

Rosen, T., et al. "Decreased Psychological Well-Being in Adult Patients with Growth Hormone Deficiency." *Clinical Endocrinology* 40 (1994): 111-16.

Rosen, T., and B-A. Bengtssön. "Premature Mortality Due to Cardiovascular Disease in Hypopituitarism." *Lancet* 336 (1990): 285-88.

Rosen, T., I. Bosaeus, J. Tolli, G. Lindstedt, and B-A. Bengtssön. "Increased Body Fat Mass and Decreased Extracellular Fluid Volume in Adults with Growth Hormone Deficiency." *Clinical Endocrinology* 38 (1993): 63-71.

Rosen, T., G. Johannson, and B-A. Bengtssön. "Consequences of Growth Hormone Deficiency in Adults, and Effects of Growth Hormone Replacement Therapy." *Acta Paediatrica* suppl. 399 (1994): 21-24.

Rosenbaum, M., J.M. Gertner, and R. Leibel, R. "Effects of Systemic Growth Hormone Administration on Regional Adipose Tissue Distribution and Metabolism in GH-Deficient Children." *Journal of Clinical Endocrinology and Metabolism* 69 (1989): 1274-81.

Rubin, C.D. "Southwestern Internal Medicine Conference: Growth Hormone--Aging and Osteoporosis." *American Journal of Medical Science* 305, no.2 (1993): 120-29.

Rudling, M., et al. "Importance of Growth Hormone for the Induction of Hepatic Low Density lipoprotein Receptors." *Proceedings of the National Academy of Sciences USA* 89 (August 1992): 6983-87.

Rudman, D. "Growth Hormone, Body Composition, and Aging." *Journal of the American Geriatrics Society* 33 (1965): 800-07.

Rudman, D. "Impaired Growth Hormone Secretion in the Adult Population: Relation to Age and Adiposity." *Journal of Clinical Investigation* 67 (1981): 1361-69.

Rudman, D., A.G. Feller, L. Cohn, K.R. Shetty, and I.W. Rudman. "Effects of Human Growth Hormone on Body Composition in Elderly Men." *Hormone Research* 6, suppl. 1 (1991): 73-81.

Rudman, D., et al. "Effects of Human Growth Hormone in Men over 60 Years Old." *New England Journal of Medicine* 323 (1990): 1-6.

Rudman, D., et al. "Relations of Endogenous Anabolic Hormones and Physical Activity to Bone Mineral Density and Lean Body Mass in Elderly Men." *Clinical Endocrinology* 40 (1994): 653-61.

Russel-Jones, D.L. "The Effects of Growth Hormone on Protein Metabolism in Adult Growth Hormone Deficient Patients." *Clinical Endocrinology* 38 (1993): 427-31.

Russel-Jones, D.L., A.J. Weissberger, S.B. Gowes, J.M. Kelly, M. Thomason, A.M. Umbleby, R.H. Jones, and P.H. Sonksen. "The Effect of Growth Hormone Replacement On Serum Lipid, Lipoproteins, Apolipoproteins, and Cholesterol Precursors in Adult Growth Hormone Deficiency Patients." *Clin Endocrinol* 41: 345-350, April 1994.

Salomon, F., R.C. Cuneo, R. Hesp, and P.H. Sonksen. "The Effects of Treatment with Recombinant Human Growth Hormone on Body Composition and Metabolism in Adults with Growth Hormone Deficiency." *New England Journal of Medicine* 321 (1989): 1797-803.

Salva, P.S., and G.E. Bacon. "Public Interest in Human Growth Hormone Therapy" (letter). *Western Journal of Medicine* 155, no.4 (October 1991): 428.

Sartorio, A., E. Molinari, G. Riva, A. Conti, F. Morabitom and G. Falia. "Growth Hormone Treatment in Adults with Childhood Onset Growth Hormone Deficiency: Effects on Psychological Capabilities." *Hormone Research* 44, no. 1 (1995): 6-11

Savard, P. "Growth Factors and Rejuvenation: General Overview of the Therapeutical Uses of Ghs and Their Market." Paper presented at the Third International Conference on Aging Medicine and Biomedical Technology, Las Vegas, Nevada, December 9-11, 1995. Schambelan, M., K. Mulligan, C. Grunfeld, E.S. Daar, A. LaMarca, D.P. Kotler, J. Wang, S.A. Bozzette, and J.B. Breitmeyer. "Recombinant Human Growth Hormone in Patients With HIV-Associated Wasting. A Randomized, Placebo-Controlled Trial. Serostim Study Group. *Ann Intern Med* 125(11):873-882, December 1996.

Shetty, K.R., and E.H. Duthie, Jr. "Anterior Pituitary Function and Growth Hormone Use in the Elderly." *Encocrinology and Metabolism Clinics of North America* 24, no.2 (1995): 213-31.

Shinobe M., T. Sanaka, H. Nihei, and N. Gugino. "IGF-1/IGFBP-1 As An Index For Discrimination Between Responder and Nonresponder to Recombinant Human Growth Hormone In Malnourished Uremic Patients On Hemodialysis." *Nephron* 77(1):29-36, 1997.

Snyder, D., L.D. Underwood, and D.R. Clammons. "Persistent Lypolytic Effect of Exogenous Growth Hormone During Caloric Restriction." *American Journal of Medicine* 98 (1995): 129-34.

Sonksen, P.H. "Replacement Therapy in Hypothalamo-Pituitary Insufficiency After Childhood: Management in the Adult." *Hormone Research* 33, suppl. 4 (1990): 45-51.

Sonntag, W.E. et al "Decreases in Cerebral Microvasculature with Age Are Associated with the Decline in Growth Hormone and Insulin-like Growth Factor 1." *Endocrinology* 34 (1982): 163-68.

Sonntag, W.E., et al. "Moderate Caloric Restriction Alters the Subcellular Distribution of Somatostatin mRNA and Increases Growth Hormone Pulse Amplitude in Aged Animals." *Neuroendocrinology* 61, no. 5 (1995): 601-08.

Takagi, K., T. Tashiro, Y. Mashima, H. Yamamori, K. Okui, and I. Ito. "The Effect of Human Growth Hormone on Protein Metabolism in the Surgically Stressed State" (in Japanese). *Nippon-Geka-Gakkai-Zasshi* 92, no. 11 (November 1991): 1545-51.

Valcavi, R., O. Gaddi, M. Zini, M. Lavicol, U. Mellino, and I. Portioli. "Cardiac Performance and Mass in Adults with Hypopituitarism: Effects of One Year of Growth Hormone Treatment." *Journal of Clinical Endocrinology and Metabolism* 80, no. 2 (1995): 695 ff.

Van Cauter, E., et al. "Simultaneous Stimulation of Slow Wave Sleep and Growth Hormone Secretion by Gamma-Hydrotbutyrate in Normal Young Men." *Journal of Clinical Investigation* 100, No. 3 (1997): 745-53.

Vergani, G., A. Mayerhofer, and A. Bartke. "Acute Effects of Human Growth Hormone on Liver Cells in Vitro: A Comparison with Livers of Mice Transgenic for Human Growth Hormone." *Tissue-Cell.* 23, no. 5 (1991): 607-12.

Verhelst, J., R. Abs, M. Vandewegh, J. Mockel, J.J. Legros, G. Copinschi, C. Mahler, C. Mahler, B. Velkeniers, L. Vanhaelst, A. Van Aelst, D. De Rijdt, A. Stevenaert, and A. Beckers. "Two Years of Replacement Therapy in Adults With Growth Hormone Deficiency." *Clin Endocrinol (Oxf)* 47(4):485-494, October 1997.

Voerman, B.J. "Effects of Human Growth Hormone in Critically Placebo-Controlled Trial." *Critical Care Medicine* 23, no. 4 (1995): 665-73.

Vreeland, L. "The Drug of the Decade?" *Ladies Home Journal,* October 1990, 91-92.

Walford, R.L. *The 120-Year Diet.* New York: Simon and Schuster, 1986.

Walker, R.F., G.C. Ness, Z. Zhao, and B.B. Bercu. "Effects of Stimulated Growth Hormone Secretion on Age-Related Changes in Plasma Cholesterol and Hepatic Low Density Lipoprotein Messenger RNA Concentrations." *Mechanisms of Ageing and Development* 73, no. 3 (September 1994): 215-26.

Warwick D.J., D.B. Lowrie, and P.J. Cole. "Growth Hormone Activation of Human Monocytes for Superoxide Production But Not Tumor Necrosis Factor Production, Cell Adherence, or Action Against Mycobacterium Tuberculosis." *Infection andImmunology* 63, no. 11 (November 1995): 4312-16.

Weigent, D.A., and J.E. Blalock. "Immunoreactive Growth Hormone-Releasing Hormone in Rat Leukocytes." *Journal of Neuroimmunology* 29 (1990): 1-13.

Weindruch, R. "Caloric Restriction and Aging." *Scientific American,* January 1966: 46-52.

Weindruch, R., and R.L. Walford. *The Retardation of Aging and Dietary Restriction.* New York: Charles C. Thomas, 1988.

Weiss, R. "A Shot at Youth." *American Health*, November-December 1993.

Whitehead, et al. "Growth Hormone Treatment of Adults with Growth Hormone Deficiency: Results of a 13-Month Placebo Controlled Cross-Over Study." *Clinical Endocrinology* 36 (1992): 45-52.

Yang, R., S. Bunting, N. Gillett, R. Clark, and H. Jin. "Growth Hormone Improves Cardiac Performance in Experimental Heart Failure." *Circulation* 92 (1995): 262-67.

Yang, R., S. Bunting, N. Gillett, R.G. Clark, and H. Jin. "Effects of Growth Hormone In Rats With Postinfarction Left Ventricular Dysfunction." *Cardiovasc Drugs Ther* 9(1):125-131, February 1995.

Ziegler, T.R., J.M. Lazarus, L.S. Young, R. Hakim, and D.W. Wilmore. "Effects of Recombinant Human Growth Hormone in Adults Receiving Maintenance Hemodialysis." *Journal of the American Society of Nephrology* 2, no. 6 (1991):1130-5.

Section IV: Other Hormones

Althaus, B.U., J.J. Staub, A. Ryff-De Leche, A. Oberhansli, and H.B. Stahelin. "LDL/HDL Changes in Subclinical Hypothyroidism: Possible Risk Factors For Coronary Heart Disease." *Clin Endocrinol* 28:157-163, February, 1988.

Andrews, W.C. "Continuous Combined Estrogen/Progestin Hormone Replacement Therapy." *Hospital Medicine*, Supplement (November 1995): 1-11.

Aver S., A.S. Dobs, A.W. Meikle, R.P. Allen, S.W. Sanders, and N.A. Mazer. "Improvement of Sexual Function in Testosterone Deficient Men Treated For One Year With a Permeation Enhanced Testosterone Trandermal System." *J Urol* 155(5):1604-1608, May 1996.

Baker, B. "Estrogen May Be Effective for Stroke Reduction." *Family Practice News*, November 1, 1995, 16.

Barnes, B. Hypothyroidism: *The Unsuspected Illness*. New York: Harper Collins, 1976.

Barret-Connor, E., K.T. Khaw, and S.S. Yen. "A Prospective Study of Dehydroepiand-rosterone Sulfate, Mortality and Cardiovascular Disease." *N Eng J Med* 315 (24):1519-1524, December 1986.

Brody, J.E. "Experimental Evidence Is Lacking for Melatonin As Cure-All." *New York Times*, September 27, 1995, C9.

Borek, Carmia, Ph.D., *Maximize Your Health-Span with Antioxidants*. Keats Publishing, Connecticut, 1995, pp13-20.

Cleary, M.P. "The Antiobesity Effect of Dehydroepiandrosterone in Rats." *Proc Soc Exp Biol Med* 196(1):8-16, January 1991.

Coles, Stephen, M.D. "CoQ-10 and Life Span Extension." *Journal of Longevity Research* Vol. 1, No. 5, 1995.

Davison, R., P. Koets, W.G. Snow, and L.G. Gabrielson. "Effects of Delta 5 Pregnenolone in Rheumatoid Arthritis." *Arch Int Med* 85:365-388, 1950.

Dawson, D., and N. Encel. "Melatonin and Sleep in Humans." *J Pineal Res* 15(1): 1-12, August 1993.

Ditkoff, E.C., W.G. Crary, M. Cristo, et al. "Estrogen Improves Psychological Function in Asymptomatic Postmenopausal Women." *Obstetrics and Gynecology* 78, no. 6 (December 1991): 991-95.

Dollins, A.B., I.V. Zhdanova, R.J. Wurtman, H.J. Lynch, and M.H. Deng. "Effect of Inducing Nocturnal Serum Melatonin Concentrations in Daytime On Sleep, Mood, Body Temperature, and Performance." *Proc Natl Acad Sci USA* 91: 1834-1828, March 1994.

Ettinger, B., G.D. Friedman, T. Bush, and C.P. Quesenberry. "Reduced Mortality Associated With Long-Term Post-Menopausal Estrogen Therapy." *Obstet Gynecol* 87(1):6-12, January 1996.

Flood, J.F., J.E. Morley, and E. Roberts. "Pregnenolone Sulfate Enhances Post-Training Memory Processes When Injected in Very Low Doses Into Limbic System Structures: The Amygdala Is By Far the Most Sensitive." *Proc Natl Acad Sci USA* 92(23):10806-108010, November 1995.

Ford, G. *Listening to Your Hormones*. Rocklin, California: Prima Publishing, 1996.

Gambrel, R.D., R.C. Maier, and B.I. Sanders. "Decreased Incidence of Breast Cancer in Postmenopausal Estrogen-Progesterone Users." *Obstet Gynecol* 62(4):435- 443, October 1983.

Guth, L., Z. Zhang, and E. Roberts. "Key Role For Pregnenolone in Combination Therapy That Promotes Recovery After Spinal Cord Injury." *Proc Natl Acad Sci USA* 91:12308-312, December, 1994.

Hargrove, J.T., W.S. Maxson, A.C. Wentz, and L.S. Burnett. "Menopausal Hormone Replacement Therapy With Continuous Daily Oral Micronized Estradiol and Progrestrone." *Obstet Gynecol* 73:606-612, April 1989.

Hendler, S.S. *The Complete Guide to Anti-Aging Nutrients*. Simon & Schuster, New York, 1984, p. 88.

Hobbs, C.J., et al. "Testosterone Administration Increases Insulin-Like Growth Factor-1 Levels in Normal Men." *Journal of Clinical Endocrinology and Metabolism* 77 (1993):776-779.

Irwin, M., A. Mascovitch, J.C. Gillin, R. Willoughby, J. Pike, and T.L. Smith. "Partial Sleep Deprivation Reduces Natural Killer Cell Activity in Humans." *Psychosom Med* 56(6):493-498, November 1994.

Iseri, L.T., et al. "Magnesium Therapy for Intractable Ventricular Tachyarrhythmias in Noromagnesemic Patients." *Western Journal of Medicine* 139 (1983): 823.

Kalimi, M., and W. Regelson. *The Biologic Role of Dehydroepiandrosterone*. New York: Walter de Gruyter, 1990.

Kaiser, F.E., S.P. Viosca, J.E. Marley, A.D. Mooradian, S.S. Davis, and S.G. Korenman. "Impotence and Aging: Clinical and Hormonal Factors." *J Am Geriatr Soc* 36(6):511-519, June 1988.

Kaiser, F., and J.E. Morley. "Gonadotropins, Testosterone and the Aging Male." *Neuro Aging* 15:559-563, July 1994.

Klatz, R.M. and R. Goldman. *Stopping the Clock*. New Canaan, CT: Keats Publishing 1996.

Klein, I. "Thyroid Hormone and the Cardiovascular System." *Am J Med* 88(6):631-637, 1990.

Lee, J.R. Natural Progesterone: *The Multiple Roles of a Remarkable Hormone*. Sebastopol, Calif.: BLL Publishing, 1993.

Lissoni P., S. Barni, G. Tancini, A. Ardizzoia, F. Rovelli, M. Cazzaniga, F. Brivio, A. Piperno, R. Aldeghi, D. Fossati, et al. "Immunotherapy With Subcutaneous Low-Dose Interleukin-2 and the Pineal Indole Melatonin as a New Effective Therapy in Advanced Cancers of the Digestive Tract." *Br J Cancer* 67(6): 1404-1407, June 1993.

Marin, P. "Testosterone and Regional Fat Distribution." *Obesity Res* 3 Suppl. 4: 609S, November 1995.

Mohr, P.E., D.Y. Wang, W.M. Gregory, M.A. Richards, and I.S. Fentiman. "Serum Progesterone and Prognosis in Operable Breast Cancer." *Br J Cancer* 73(12):1552-1555, June 1996.

Meziane, H., C. Mathis, S.M.Paul, and A. Ungerer. "The Neurosteroid Pregnenolone Sulfate Reduces Learning Deficits Induced By Appetitive Learning Task." *Psychopharmacology (Berl)* 126(4):323-330, August 1996.

Morales, A.J., J.J. Nolan, J.C. Nelson, and S.S. Yen. "Effects of Replacement Dose of Dehydroepiandrosterone in Men and Women of Advancing Age." *J Clin Endocrin Metab* 78(6):1360-1367, June 1994.

Nyholm, H.C., I.J. Christensen, and A.L. Nielsen. "The Prognostic Significance of Progesterone Receptor Level in Endometrial Cancer." Ugeskr Laeger 159(5): 604, January 1997.

Peat, R. "Thyroid: Misconceptions.: *Townsend Letter for Doctors* November 1993 1120-22.

PEPI Trial. (The Writing Group for the PEPI Trial.) "Effects of Estrogen or Estrogen/Progestin Regimens On Heart Disease Risk Factors in Postmenopausal Women. *J Am Med Assoc* 273:199-208, February 1995.

PEPI Trial. (The Writing Group for the PEPI Trial.) "Effects of Hormone Replacement Therapy On Endometrial Histology in Postmenopausal Women." *J Am Med Assoc* 275(5):370-375, February 1996.

Pierpaoli, W., and W. Regelson. *The Melatonin Miracle*. New York: Simon and Schuster, 1995.

Pierpaoli, W., and W. Regelson. "Pineal Control of Aging: Effect of Melatonin and Pineal Grafting on Aging Mice." *Proc Natl Acad Sci USA* 94:787-791, January 1994.

Pierpaoli, W., D. Bulian, A. Dall'Ara, B. Marchetti, F. Gallo, M.C. Morale, C. Tirolo, and N. Testa. "Circadian Melatonin and Young-to-Old Pineal Grafting Postpone Aging and Maintain Juvenile Conditions of Reproductive Functions in Mice and Rats." *Exp Gerontol* 32(4-5):587-602, July 1997.

Phillips, G.B., B.H. Pinkernell, and T.Y. Jing. "The Association of Hypotestosteronemia With Coronary Artery Disease in Men." *Arterioscler Thromb* 14:701-706, November 1994.

Pincus, G. and H. Hoagland. "Effects of Administered Pregnenolone on Fatiguing Psychomotor Performances." *J Aviat Med* 15:98-115, 1945.

Pincus, G. and H. Hoagland. "Effects of Industrial Production of the Administration of Delta 5 Pregnenolone to Factory Workers." *Psychosomatic Med* 7:342-346, 1945.

Prior, J.C. "Progesterone As a Bone-Trophic Hormone." *Endocrine Revs* 11:386-398, May 1990.

Regelson, W., and C. Coleman. *The Superhormone Promise* New York: Simon and Schuster, 1996.

Reiter, R.J., D.X. Tan, B. Poeggeler, A. Menendez-Pelaez, L.D. Chen, and S. Saarela. "Melatonin As a Free Radical Scavenger: Implications For Aging and Age-Related Diseases." *Ann NY Acad Sci* 719:1-12, May 1994.

Reiter, R.J. "Pineal Functioning During Aging: Attenuation of the Melatonin Rhythm and Its Neurobiological Consequences." *Acta Neurobiol Exp* (Warsz) 54:31-39, 1994.

Roberts, G. "Dehydroepiandrosterone (DHEA) and it Sulfate (DHEAS) As Neural Facilitators: Effects On Brain Tissue in Culture and On Memory in Young and Old Mice. Acylic GMP hypothesis of Action of DHEA and DHEAS in Nervous System and Other Tissues." *The Biologic Role of Dehydroepiandrosterone* (DHEA), M. Kalimi and W. Regelson, eds, New York: Walter de Gruyter, 1990.

Roy, J.A., C.A. Sawka, and K.I. Pritchard. "Hormone Replacement Therapy in Women With Breast Cancer. Do the Risks Outweigh the Benefits?" *J Clin Oncol* 14(3): 997-1006, March 1996.

Rozencwaig, R., B.R. Grad, and J. Ochoa. "The Role of Melatonin and Seratonin in Aging." *Medical Hypotheses* 23, no. 4 (August 1987): 337.

Schwartz, J. R., R. Freeman, and W. Frishman. "Clinical Pharmacology of Estrogens: Cardiovascular Actions and Cardioprotective Benefits of Replacement Therapy in Postmenopausal Women." *J Clin Pharmacol* 35(3): 1-16, 35(3):314-329, January, March 1995.

Shealy, N.C. DHEA: *The Youth and Health Hormone*. New Canaan: Keats Publishing Inc, 1996.

Sherwin, B.B. "Estrogen and/or Androgen Replacement Therapy and Cognitive Functioning in Surgically Menopausal Women." *Psychoneuroendocrinology* 13(4):345-357, 1988.

Sherwin, B.B. "Sex Hormones and Psychological Functioning in Postmenopausal Women." *Exp Gerontol* 29:423-430, May 1994.

Tang, M.X., D. Jacobs, Y. Stern, K. Marder, P. Schofield, B. Gurland, H. Andrews, and R. Mayeux. "Effect of Oestrogen During Menopause on Risk and Age at Onset of Alzheimer's Disease." *Lancet* 348:429-432, August 1996.

Weideger P. Menstruation and Menopause: *The Physiology and Psychology, the Myth and the Reality*. New York: Alfred A. Knopf, 1976.

Weiss, N.S. "Health Consequences of Short-and Long-Term Postmenopausal Hormone Therapy." *Clin Chem* 42(8 Pt 2):1342-1344, August 1996.

Wolkowitz, O.M., V.I. Reus, E. Roberts, F. Manfredi, T. Chan, W.J. Raum, S. Ormiston, R. Johnson, J. Canick, L. Brizendine, and H. Weingartner. "Dehydroepiandrosterone (DHEA) Treatment of Depression." *Biol Psychiatry* 41(3):311-318, February 1997.

Zhdanova, I.V., R.J. Wurtman, H.J. Lynch, J.R. Ives, A.B. Dollins, C. Morabito, J.K. Matheson, and D.L. Schomer. "Sleep-Inducing Effects of Low Doses of Melatonin Ingested in the Evening." *Clin Pharmacol Ther* 57:552-558, May 1995.

Zubialde, J.P., F. Lawler, and N. Clemenson. "Estimated Gains in Life Expectancy With Use of Postmenopausal Estrogen Therapy: A Decision Analysis." *J Fam Prac* 36:271-289, March 1993.

Section V: Antioxidants, Minerals, & Other Supplements

Abraham, G.E., "Nutritional Factors in the Etiology of the Premenstrual Tension Syndromes." *Journal of Reproductive Medicine*, 1983, 28:446-464, cited in *Formulas for Life*, p. 168.

Anderson, R.A., et al. "Chromium Supplementation of Human Subjects: Effects on Glucose, Insulin, and Lipid Variables." 1983, 32: 894-899, cited in Kronhausen, Eberhard, Ed.D., and Phyllis Kronhausen, Ed.D., with Harry B. Demopoulos, M.D., *Formulas For Life*, William Morrow, New York, 1989, p. 172.

Balch, J.F., and Balch P.A. *Prescription for Nutritional Healing*. New York: Avery Publishing, 1990.

Borek, Carmia. Ph.D., *Maximize Your Health Span with Antioxidants*. Keats Publishing, New Canaan, Conn., 1995 p 63.

Brown, D.J. "Ginkgo Biloba--Old and New: Part II." *Let's Live* May 1992.

Clark, L.C., G.F. Combs Jr., C.L. Smith, and J.R. Taylor. "Effects of Selenium Supplementation For Cancer Prevention in Patients With Carcinoma of the Skin: A Randomized Controlled Trial. Nutritional Prevention of Cancer Study Group." *J Am Med Assoc* 276(24):1957-1963, December 1996.

Dyckner, T., and P.O Wester, "Effect of Magnesium on Blood Pressure." *British Medical Journal* 286 (1983): 1847.

Ford, Norman. *Lifestyle for Longevity*. Para Research, Gloucester, Mass. 1984: 82-83.

Frankel, E.N., J. Kanner, J.B. German, E. Parks, and J.E. Kinsella. "Inhibition of Oxidation of Human Low-Density Lipoprotein by Phenolic Substances in Red Wine." *Lancet* 341:454-457, February 1993.

Hansen, *C. Grape Seed Extract: Procyanidolic Oligomers* (PCP). New York: Healing Wisdom Publications, 1995.

Kamikawa, T., A. Kobayashi, T. Yamashita, H. Hayashi, and N. Yamazaki. "Effects of Coenzyme Q-10 On Exercise Tolerance in Chronic Stable Angina Pectoris." *Am J Cardiol* 56(4):247-251, August 1985.

Kemnitz, J.W., E.B. Roecker, R. Weindruch, D.R. Elson, S.T. Baum, and R.N. Berman. "Dietary Restriction Increases Insulin Sensitivity and Lowers Blood Glucose in Rhesus Monkeys." Am J Physiol 266(4 Pt 1):E540-547, April 1994.

Le Bars, P.L., M.M. Datz, N. Berman, T.M. Itil, A.M. Freedman, and A.F. Schatzberg. "A Placebo-Controlled, Double-Blind, Randomized Trial of an Extract of Ginkgo Biloba for Dementia. North American Egb Study Group." *JAMA* Oct. 22;278(16): 1327-1332, October 1997.

Lee, William H. Coenzyme Q-10: *Is it Our New Fountain of Youth?* New Canaan, Conn.: Keats Publishing, 1987.

Lesourd, B. "Nutrition and Immunity in the Elderly: Modification of Immune Responses With Nutritional Treatment." *Am J Clin Nutr* 66(2):478S-484S, August 1997.

Levine, S.A., and P.M. Kidd. *Antioxidant Adaptation: Its Role in Free Radical Pathology* Biocurrents Division, Allergy Research Group, San Leandro (1986): 241-242.

"Life Extension Update: CoQ-10 Reduces Surgical Complications." *Life Extension Magazine.* (March 1, 1995): 4-5.

Lolic, M.M., G. Fiskum, and R.E. Rosenthal. "Neuroprotective Effects of Acetyl-L-Carnitine After Stroke in Rats." *Ann Emerg Med* June 29(6):758-765, June 1997.

Marchesini, G., et al. Anticatabolic Effect of Branched-Chain Amino Acid-Enriched *Solutions in Patients With Liver Cirrhosis. Hepatology.* 2:420-425, 1982.

Mesones, H.L. "Coenzyme Q-10 in Psychiatry." *Acta Psiquiatr Psicol Am Lat* 40(3): 207-210, September 1994.

Mowrey, D.B. *Herbal Tonic Therapies* New Canaan, Con.: Keats Publishing, 1993.

Murray, F. *Ginkgo Biloba: the Amazing 200 Million-Year-Old Healer.* New Canaan, Conn.: Keats Publishing, 1993.

Paolisso, G., A. Gambardella, D. Giugliano, D. Galzerano, L. Amato, C. Volpe, V. Balbi, M. Varricchio, and F. D'Onofrio. "Chronic Intake of Pharmacological Doses of Vitamin E might be useful in the Therapy of Elderly Patients With Coronary Heart Disease." *Am J Clin Nutr* 81:848-852, April 1995.

Perrig, G., P. Perrig, and H.B. Stahelin. "The Relations Between Antioxidants and Memory Performance in the Old and Very Old." *J Am Geriatr Soc* 45(6):718-724, June 1997.

Riales, R., and M.J. Albrink. "Effect of Chromium Chloride Supplementation on Glucose Tolerance and Serum Lipids Including High-Density Lipoprotein of Adult Men." *American Journal of Clinical Nutrition.* 34 (1981):2670-2678.

Salonen, J.T., et al. "Risk of Cancer in Relation to Serum Concentrations of Selenium and Vitamins A and E: Matched CSE Control Analysis of Prospective Data." *British Medical Journal* 290 (1985): 417.

Scharrer, A., and M. Ober. "Anthocyanosides in the Treatment of Retinopathies." Klin Monatsble Augenheilkd 178:386-389, May 1981.

Schmuck, A. A. Ravel, C. Coudray, J. Alary, A. Franco, and A.M. Roussel. "Antioxidant Vitamins in Hospitalized Elderly Patients: Analysed Dietary Intakes and Biochemical Status." *Eur J Clin Nutr* 50(7):473-478, July 1996.

Sonntag, W.E., J.E. Lenham, and R.L. Ingram. "Effects of Aging and Dietary Restriction on Tissue Protein Synthesis: Relationship to Plasma Insulin-Like Growth Factor-1." *J Gerontol* 47(5):B159-163, September 1992.

Tronnier, H. "Clinical-Pharmacological Studies on the Effect of an Extract From Ginkgo Biloba L in the Post thrombotic Syndrome." *Arzneimittelforschung* 18(5):551- 554, May 1968.

Turturro, A., K. Blank, D. Murasko, and R. Hart. "Mechanisms of Caloric Restriction Affecting Aging and Disease." *Ann NY Acad Sci* 719:159-170, May 1994.

Turlapaty, P.D., and B.M. Altura. "Magnesium Deficiency Produces Spasms of Coronary Arteries: Relationship to Etiology of Sudden Death Ischemic Heart Disease." *Science* 208 (1980): 198.

Weitbrecht, W.V., and W. Jansen. "Double-Blind and Comparative (Ginkgo Biloba vs. Placebo) Therapeutic Study in Geriatric Patients With Primary Degenerative Dementia--A Preliminary Evaluation." *Effects of Ginkgo Biloba Extract on Organic Cerebral Impairment.* A. Agnoli, et al, eds. London: Eurotext Ltd, 1985.

Section VI: Conclusion

Bailey, A.R., R.G. Smith, and G. Leng. "The Nonpeptide Growth Hormone Secretogogue, Mk00677, Activates Hypothalamic Arcuate Nucleus Neurons in Vivo." *J Neuroendocrinol* 10(2):111-118, February 1998.

Ball, S.E., F.M. Gibson, S. Rizzo, J.A. Tooze, J.C. Marsh, and E.C. Gordon-Smith. "Progressive Telomere Shortening in Aplastic Anemia."

Bellone, J., et al. "Growth Hormone-Releasing Activity of Hexarelin, a New Synthetic Hexapeptide, Before and During Puberty." *Journal of Clinical Endocrinology and Metabolism* 80, no. 4 (1994): 1090-94.

Biochemistry (Moscow). Special Issue. Telomere, Telomerase, *Cancer And Aging.* Volume 62, no. 11 (1997).

Blackburn, E.H. "The Telomere and Telomerase: Nucleic Acid-Protein Complexes Acting in a Telomere Homeostasis System. *A Review. Biochemistry (Moscow),*Volume 62, no. 11 (1997): 1196.

Bodnar, A.G., M. Ouellette, M. Frolkis, S.E. Holt, C.P. Chiu, G.B. Morin, C.B. Harley J. Shay, S. Lichsteiner, and W.E. Wright. "Extension of Life-Span by Introduction of Telomerase Into Normal Human Cells." *Science* 279(5349):349-352, January 1998.

Bowers, C.Y. "Gh Releasing Peptides--Structure and Kinetics." *Journal of Pediatric Endocrinology* 6, no. 1 (1993): 21-31.

Bowers, C.Y. "An Overview of the GH Releasing Peptides (GHRPs), Growth Hormone Secretagogues" (abstract). Paper presented at Serano Symposia USA, December 8-11, 1994.

Bowers, C.Y., D.K. Alster, and J.M. Frentz. "The Growth Hormone-Releasing Activity of a Synthetic Hexapeptide in Normal Men and Short Statured Children After Oral Administration." *Journal of Clinical Endocrinology and Metabolism* 74 (1992): 292-98.

Bowers, C.Y., G.A. Reynolds, D. Durham, et al. "Growth Hormone (GH)-Releasing Peptide Stimulates GH Release in Normal Men and Acts Synergistically with GH-Releasing Hormone." *Journal of Clinical Endocrinology and Metabolism* 70, no. 4 (1994): 975-82.

Brien, T.P., B.V. Kallakury, C.V. Lowry, R.A. Ambros, P.J. Muraca, J.H. Falfetano and J.S Ross. "Telomerase Activity in Benign Endometrium and Endometrial Carcinoma." *Cancer Res* 57(13):2760-2764, July 1997.

Bryan, T.M., R.R. Reddel. "Telomere Dynamics and Telomerase Activity in in Vitro Immortalized Human Cells." *Eur J Cancer* 33(5):767-773, April 1997.

Camanni, F. E. Ghigo, and E. Arvat. "Growth Hormone-Releasing Peptides and Their Analogs." *Front Neuroendocrinol* 19(1):47-72, January 1998.

Camanni, F., E. Ghigo, and E. Arvat. "Growth Hormone-Releasing Peptides." *Euro J Endocrinol* 136(5): 445-460, May 1997.

Ehrenstein, D. "Immortality Gene Discovered." *Science* 279:177, January 1998.

Ghigo, E., E. Arvat, L. Gianotte, et al. Growth Hormone-Releasing Activity of Hexarelin, A New Synthetic Hexapeptide, After Intravenous Subcutaneous, Intranasal, and Oral Administration in Man." *Journal of Clinical Endocrinology and Metabolism* 78, no. 3 (1994):693-98.

Kemnitz, J.W., E.B. Roecker, R. Weindruch, D.R. Elson, S.T. Baum, and R.N. Bergman. "Dietary Restriction Increases Insulin Sensitivity and Lowers Blood Glucose in Rhesus Monkeys." *Am J Physiol* 266(4 Pt 1):E540-547, April 1994.

Kinouchi, Y., N. Hieatashi, M. Chida, F. Nagashima, S. Takagi, H. Mackawa, and T. Toyota. "Telomer Shortening in the Colonic Mucosa of Patients With Ulcerative Colitis." *J Gastroenterol* 33(3):343-348, June 1998.

Metcalfe, J.A., J. Parkhill, L. Campbell, M. Stacey, P. Biggs, P.J. Byrd, and M.R. Taylor. "Accelerated Telomere Shortening in Ataxia Telangiectasia." *Natr Genetics* 13(3):350, July 1996.

Parkes, T.L., A.J. Elia, D. Dickenson, A.J. Hilliker, J.P. Phillips, and G.L. Boulianne. "Extension of Drosophila Lifespan by Overexpression of Human SOD1 in Motorneurons." *Nat Genet* 19(2):171-174, 1998.

Stokkan, K.A., R.J. Reiter, K.O.Nonaka, A. Lerchl, B.P. Yu, and M.K. Vaughan. "Food Restriction Retards Aging of the Pineal Gland." *Brain Res* 545(102):66-72, April 1991.

Smith, R.G., et al. "Modulation of Pulsatile GH Release Through a Novel Receptor in Hypothalamus and Pituitary Gland." Journal of *Molecular Endocrinology* 1, no. 10 (1996): 261-86.

Smith, Roy, G., Kang Cheng, William R. Schoen, et al. "A Nonpeptidyl Growth Hormone Secretagogue." *Science* 260 (June 11, 1993): 1640-43.

Tuilpakov, A.N., et al. "Growth Hormone (GH)-Releasing Effects of Synthetic Peptide GH-Releasing Peptide-2 and GH-Releasing Hormone in Children with GH Insufficiency and Idiopathic Short Stature." *Metabolism* 44, no. 9 (September 1996): 1199-1204.

Valetto, M.R., et al. *Reproducibility of the Growth Hormone Response to Stimulation With Growth Hormone-Releasing Hormone Plus Arginine During Lifespan.* European Journal of Endocrinology. 135(5):568-572, 1996.

Waldholz, M. "Merck Develops Type of Human Growth Drug." *Wall Street Journal* June 11, 1993.

Weindruch, R., R.L. Walford, S. Fligiel, and D. Guthrie. "The Retardation of Aging in Mice by Dietary Restriction: Longevity, Cancer, Immunity and Lifetime Energy Intake." *J Nutr* 116(4):641-654, April 1986.

Index

Index

hair, 11, 40, 51, 65, 109-111, 172, 174, 175, 186, 192, 216, 250

Harmon, Dr. Denham, 300

Hayflick, Dr. Leonard, 37, 38, 39, 265, 266, 299, 300, 309

Hayflick limit theory, 37

HDL, 115, 116, 175, 176, 224, 322

healing, 50, 65, 123, 128, 129, 131, 302, 307, 314, 328, 329

heart, 29, 31, 37, 38, 50, 60, 62, 83, 94, 98, 103, 106, 111, 113-117,
        119, 132, 135, 175, 176, 182, 190, 191, 202, 216,
        218, 220, 222-226, 247, 252, 271, 304, 314, 321,
        322, 325, 330, 331

Heller, 183

hepatitis, 143

herpes, 143

Hertoghe, Dr. Thierry, 100, 309

HGH, 13, 17, 19, 20, 21, 45, 47, 49-64, 66-74, 76-90, 92, 94, 96-
        103, 105-129, 131-140, 144-149, 151, 152-158, 165,
        168, 169, 176, 197, 200, 202, 203, 204, 237-241,
        245-254, 261-264, 266, 270, 281, 283, 299, 301

Hill, D. E, 127, 304

histamine, 220

Hormone, 126, 199, 173, 293

Hormone Binding Globulin (SHBG), 185

hormone replacement therapy, 19, 60, 62, 63, 66, 163, 168, 170,
        174, 175, 181, 202, 249, 302, 315-317, 322, 323,
        325, 326

Human Growth Hormone, 19, 39, 42, 51, 55, 92, 121, 281, 293,
        301, 30-307, 309-312, 314-321

hydrogen peroxide, 212

hydroxyl radical, 212

hypertension, 116, 218

hypothalamus, 67-69, 76, 78, 185, 187, 200, 248, 293, 333

Epilogue

Aging as a Disease?

As we have alluded to earlier, menopause has been an established medical entity for which hormone balancing treatments have been available for many, many years. Our enhanced knowledge of this condition has led us to start using more and more natural estrogens and progesterones and we now favour those over the synthetic versions. Andropause, the decline in male hormones as we age, is now an accepted medical, clinical, treatable entity, too.

Somapause, the decline in human growth hormone and some of the other non-sexing hormones as we age, is currently not considered to be an insurable service by any medical plan that we are aware of, whether a publically or privately funded system.From a philosophical perspective it is looked on much the same way as cosmetic surgery.

We do however feel that its day is coming as more and more information becomes available with regard to human growth hormone and other hormones. Studies such as the one by Dr. Eve Van Cauter published on August 16, 2000 in the "Journal of the American Medical Association" with regard to human growth hormone decline associated with poorer sleep pattern in males as they age, are felt to bring the concept of aging as a treatable condition more into the mainstream. It is conceivable that insuring bodies at some point in the future may wish to help cover the cost of this kind of service as theoretically healthier people would have less cause to use medical assistance as those who are not as healthy as they age. For the moment, though, readers who are interested in anti-aging treatments would be well-advised to seek out physicians interested in anti-aging medicine for further advice and recommendations. A primary source for those individuals would be through the American Academy of Anti-Aging Medicine (A4M) in the U.S., or in Canada, the Canadian Longevity and Anti-Aging Academy (CLA4). Web sites that may be of interest are listed below:

http://www.cla4.com
http://www.healthandlongevitycentre.com
http://www.worldhealth.net

Dr. McLeod and Dr. White's next exciting new book dealing with everything you wanted to know about Antioxidants, entitled.

"Doctors' Secrets...The AntiOxidant Highway"

will be available in the spring of 2002.

CANADIAN LONGEVITY AND ANTI-AGING ACADEMY

A team of professionals that are dedicated to slowing the onset of degenerative diseases and promoting a healthy lifespan by utilizing the latest scientific research in the quest for longevity.

CLA4 MISSION STATEMENT

VISION: We are advancing toward a new era of increasingly powerful and sophisticated technology. The Canadian Longevity and Anti-Aging Academy, which is a non profit organization of Physicians, scientists, health researchers and interested individuals, proposes to bring the best of anti-aging therapies to Canada to allow us each to make a choice about how we age.

MISSION: Members of the Academy believe that aging and disability from degenerative disease including cardiovascular disease, cancer, diabetes and neurological deterioration is not inevitable. The Academy provides a public forum for discussion, development and promotion of medical practice, technology and therapeutics that retard or even reverse the deterioration of the human body resulting from the physiology of aging.

GOALS: To promote changes in the medical curriculum so that future physicians will be well informed in the developments in anti-aging medicine. To raise awareness among the public and to disseminate evidence based information to physicians to apply the clinical application of longevity medicine. To act as an information source for anti-aging science and to act as a liaison for government in future studies of longevity.

DISCLAIMER

The contents of this book are the opinions of the authors and may not represent the consensus of opinion of the medical profession at this time. The contents of this book are not intended to be used to treat, cure, mitigate or diagnose any medical condition. The readers should consult their doctors before embarking on any changes that could affect their health.